English Grammar Workbook

Workbook

– BASICS WORKOUT

Prof. Shrikant Prasoon

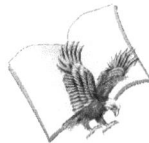

V&S PUBLISHERS

Published by:

V&S PUBLISHERS

F-2/16, Ansari road, Daryaganj, New Delhi-110002
☎ 23240026, 23240027 • *Fax:* 011-23240028
Email: info@vspublishers.com • *Website:* www.vspublishers.com

Regional Office : Hyderabad
5-1-707/1, Brij Bhawan (Beside Central Bank of India Lane)
Bank Street, Koti, Hyderabad - 500 095
☎ 040-24737290
E-mail: vspublishershyd@gmail.com

Branch Office : Mumbai
Jaywant Industrial Estate, 2nd Floor–222, Tardeo Road
Opposite Sobo Central Mall, Mumbai – 400 034
☎ 022-23510736
E-mail vspublishersmum@gmail.com

Follow us on:

All books available at **www.vspublishers.com**

Publisher's Note

V&S Publishers is proud to present another learning tool for all those wanting to improve English grammar for writing better English Today, English has become indispensable in India and abroad, as it is considered to be standard language of communication across the world. Hence, learning it has become a necessity, irrespective of age, profession, gender etc. This workbook helps you improve the language by means of practice, practice and more practice. Through 25 chapters in the book, exercises have been drawn from Parts of Speech, Nouns, Pronouns, Adjectives, Prepositions, Tenses, Direct & Indirect speech, Phrases, Idioms, and other important constituents of Grammar. For easier learning, the lessons have been grouped together and placed in chapters.

The Workbook has been designed with an aim of helping students practice the concepts using hundreds of practice questions of all types . It is a practice book aimed at mastering the concepts Do practice every day, at least one page and be on the way to good English.

Dedication

Dedicated to all those who are eager to know, learn and use English in everyday life and prefer the direct method of Learning and Teaching. I also dedicate this book to Nishi Kant Tiwari, alias Nanhejee and to Arun Kumar Ojha, alias Barā Bābu, who made the best use of tables given in the book in their classrooms.

Contents

Chapter 1

Parts of Speech

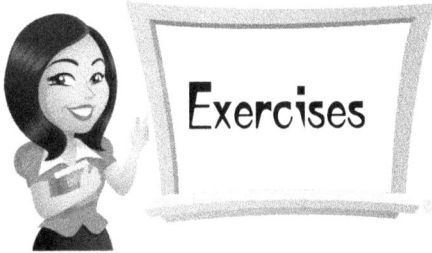

Exercises

1. Name the parts of speech of each italicised word in the following sentences, giving in each case your reason for the classification:

1.   *Still* waters run deep.
2.   He *still* lives in that house.
3.   After the storm comes the *calm.*
4.   The *after effects* of the drug are bad.
5.   It weighs about a *pound.*
6.   He told us *all* about the battle.
7.   He was only a yard *off* me.
8.   Suddenly, one of the wheels came *off.*
9.   Mohammedans *fast* in the month of Ramzan.
10. He kept the *fast* for a week.
11. He is *on* the committee.
12. Let us move *on.*
13. Sit down and rest a *while.*
14. I will watch *while* you sleep.
15. They *while* away their evenings with books and games.

Chapter 2

Nouns

Exercises

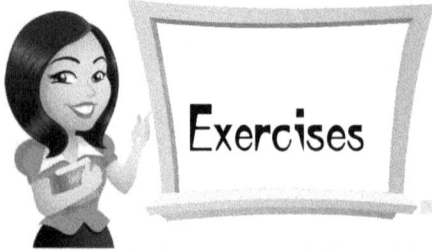

1. **Form as many sentences as you can from the table below and underline the nouns. Also specify the kind of noun in each case:**

			a good teacher.
			a famous painter.
Rahul's	brother	is	an active politician
His	sister	was	a dull worker.
My	mother	will be	a rich lawyer.
Her	father		a popular doctor.
Our	uncle		a hard worker.
Their	aunt		a smooth runner.
Your	nephew		a perfect magician.
			a pop singer.
			a great artist.
			very happy.
			very tired.
			very serious.
			very happy.
			very angry.
			seriously ill.
			extremely happy.

Number of sentences that can be formed—3927

❏   *For Example: Rahul's brother is a good teacher.*

Rahul-Proper Noun, Brother-Common Noun, Teacher—Common Noun

❏ *Rahul's brother is very happy.*

Rahul-Proper Noun, Brother-Common Noun, Happy-Abstract Noun

2. **Similarly, make as many sentences as you can from the table given below and underline the nouns. Also specify the kind of noun in each case.**

For Example: There is a <u>bridge</u> over the <u>river</u>, <u>Cauveri</u>.

Bridge and River-Common Nouns, Cauveri-Proper Noun.

Note: All the sentences in the above table begin with 'There'.

3. **Study the table given below carefully and form as many sentences as you can. Underline the nouns and also specify the type of noun in each case.**

There is	a boy	in this college.
There was	a girl	in the school.
There will be	a player	on the platform.
There is not	a doctor	in the market.
There was not	a crowd	in that street.
There will not be	a lame man	near the hall.

Note: All the sentences in the above table begin with 'There'. Also, there is one sentence of **Present Tense**, *one of the* **Past Tense** *and one of the* **Future Tense**, *and* **Positive** *in nature. Similarly, the last three sentences are also in Present Tense, Past Tense and Future Tense, but* **Negative** *in nature.*

❖❖❖

Chapter 3

Pronouns

Exercises

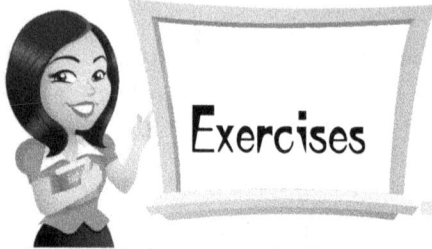

1. **Choose the correct word from each bracket and complete the sentence.**
   - ❑ We scored as many goals as (they, them).
   - ❑ Whom can I trust, if not (she, her).
   - ❑ I am one year older than (he, him).
   - ❑ I am richer than (they, them).
   - ❑ He is as good a student as (she, her)
   - ❑ The hotel (which, what) we stayed at last summer is now closed.
   - ❑ The boy (who, whom) fell off his bicycle has hurt his leg.
   - ❑ I have not seen the boy (whose, whom) suitcase was stolen.
   - ❑ Kalidasa was a great poet (who, that) wrote interesting plays.
   - ❑ Rekha is the maid (who, whom) I have employed.

2. **Join together each of the following pairs of sentences by means of a relative pronoun:**
   - ❑ Here is the book. I told you about it.
   - ❑ Did you receive the parcel? I sent the parcel yesterday.
   - ❑ Ramesh tells lies. He deserves to be punished.
   - ❑ Here is the doctor. The doctor cured me of fever.
   - ❑ This is the man. We were saved through his courage.
   - ❑ Show me the road. The road leads to the airport.
   - ❑ The boy won the first prize. You see him sitting there.
   - ❑ They heard some news. The news astonished them.
   - ❑ She spoke to the victim. The victim's arm was in a sling.
   - ❑ he conference was a success. It was held in Pune.

1. **Make as many sentences as you can using the pronouns : It, This, That, There and Here. Underline the Pronoun in each case.**

			book.
It	is	a	bag.
This			table.
That			hat.
There			mat.
Here			torch.
			chair.
			diary.
			bottle.
			ball.
			box.
			fan.
			pencil.
			lamp.
			toy.
			bell.
			bat.
			flag.
			lock.
			key.
			kite.
			ship.
			copy.
			toffee.

Note: Take one word from each column and complete a sentence, such as:

For example: It is a book.
         This is a book.
         That is a book.
         There is a book.
         Here is a book.

2. Similarly, form as many sentences as you can with the help of the pronouns: It, This, That, There given below.

			glass.
	is not/isn't	a	gun.
It			goat.
This			cage.
That			comb.
There			cow.
			clip.
			crow.
			chain.
			bulb.
			bench.
			bed.
			bicycle.
			doll.
			drum.
			dress.
			tap.
			truck.
			train.
			tray.
			pillow.
			pot.
			plate.
			lion.
			zebra.

Note: In this case, you will get only Negative Sentences.

For example: It is not/isn't a glass, or this is not/isn't a gun.

3. In the next table drawn below, you have to again form as many sentences as you can with the given pronouns, it, this, that, there and here. Take one word from each column and complete a sentence. Make all the sentences you can form with the pronoun : 'it' and then begin with 'this', 'that', 'there', and so on…

Is		a	round table?	?
	it		silver pot?	
	this		black dog?	
	that		dairy farm?	
	there		rubber stamp?	
	here		smooth blade?	
			measuring tape?	
			Sunday Magazine?	
			table tray?	
			tea stall?	
			small chair?	
			red car?	
			new gun?	
			long stick?	
			golden chain.	
			leafy tree?	
			sewing machine?	
			old skirt?	
			teaspoon?	
			rose garden?	

Note: However, in this table, all the sentences begin with 'Is', asking Questions.

*For example: Is **it** a round table? Is **this** a silver pot? Is **that** a black dog?*

And so on…

4. Make as many sentences as you can with the pronouns listed in the table given below. Select each pronoun and form as many sentences as you can. Like: It is a phone, It is a file, It is a mask, It is a register and so on…

		is a	file	?
	It		phone	
	This		mask	
	That		register	
	There		shuttle cock	
			powerful torch	
			open basket	
			musical doll	
			beautiful	
			calendar	
			sports shoe	
			chewing gum	
			big box	
			new bicycle	
			blue shirt	
			black dog	
			flying disc	
			night lamp	
			neck tie	
			sharp knife	
			round dish	

Note: However, each of the sentences that are formed above ask a Question. They may not appear so, but they can be used as Questions.

For example: It is a phone? It is a mask? It is a file?

And so on…

5. **Make as many sentences as you can with the pronouns given below. However, you must pick up one pronoun and form all the sentences and then pick up the other and form all the sentences. In this way, try making as many sentences as you can. This will enhance your vocabulary and at the same time, make you thorough with pronouns.**

			orange.
It	is		eye.
This	was	an	arm.
That			ant.
			iron.
			office.
			airbus.
			airship.
			airplane.
			ear.
			apple.
			axe.
			answer.
			inkpot.
			umbrella.
			asbestos sheet.
			aluminum plate.
			onion.
			onion salad.
			artistic article.

Note: *All the sentences formed above begin with* **Pronouns** *but have the word, 'an' instead of 'a' or 'the'. This is because they are used before words that begin with* **vowel sounds**.

6. Make as many sentences as you can with the pronouns given below.

It This That	is was	Not	An	orange. eye. arm. ant. iron. office. airbus. airship. airplane. ear. apple. axe. answer. inkpot. umbrella. asbestos sheet. aluminum plate. onion. onion salad. artistic article.

Note: All the sentences formed above have 'an' and are negative sentences.

Moreover, you can form both present and past tense types of sentences using 'is' and 'was'.

7. Form as many questions as you can with the words given below in the table.

Is	it		Orchid	?
Was	this	An	eyeball	
	that		armchair	
			anthill	
			Iron bar	
			official flat	
			airbus term	
			airship hangar	
			airdrome	
			earring	
			apple pie	
			axe	
			answer sheet	
			inkjet printer	
			atomic umbrella	
			asbestos sheet	
			iron plate	
			easy task	
			elementary	
			lesson	
			agricultural	
			product	

*Note: All the sentences formed in this case will have **question marks** at their ends and will also have **'an'** in them as they are used before words beginning with **vowel sounds**.*

8. Form as many sentences as you can with the pronouns : it, this and that.

			place.
It	is	the	house.
This	was		uniform.
That			chart.
			way.
			form.
			shop.
			sweater.
			order.
			office.
			flag.
			watch.
			street.
			shirt.
			skirt.
			case.
			coat.
			ornament.
			cooler.
			cup.

Note: All the sentences that will be formed above are both in present and past tenses and have '**the**' instead of 'a' or an 'as' they indicate some particular or definite object, or talk about a definite matter.

English Grammar Workbook

9. Form as many sentences as you can with the words given in the table below.

It This That	is was	not	the	phone book. rule. man. pen I lost. picture he gave. photo he needs. figure I drew. toffee that I want. table of the office. bed sheet I like. call I am waiting for. camera I gave you. answer. inkpot. umbrella. asbestos sheet. aluminum plate. onion. onion salad. artistic article.

Note: All the sentences formed above will have **'the'** and **'not'**, i.e., they are basically **Negative Sentences** with 'the' in them indicating some definite objects or matter.

10. Make as many sentences as you can with the pronouns, these and those and underline the pronouns.

These Those	are were	not	authentic flags. street dogs. modern houses. pet birds. rough copies. intelligent boys. house plants. rainy coats. weather charts. race horses. steel chairs. regular beggars. green trees. old pants. new maps. Indian cows. mild animals. text books. working girls. new benches. half shirts. right keys. table fans. cheap mobiles. costly computers.

Note: *Also make sure that the sentences formed from the table contain both* **Positive** *and* **Negative** *Sentences and are both in* **Present** *and* **Past Tenses***.*

For Example:

These are authentic flags.   *These were authentic flags.*
These are not authentic flags.   *These were not authentic flags.*
Those are rough copies.   *Those were rough copies.*
Those are not rough copies.   *Those were not rough copies.*

❧✦❧

❑

Chapter 4

Articles

Exercises

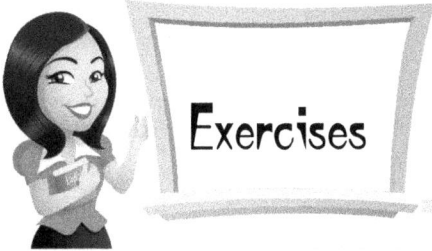

1. Supply or insert *a*, *an* or *the*, if necessary in the following sentences and rewrite them appropriately.

- ❑ Bus arrived quarter of hour late.
- ❑ Man cannot live by bread alone.
- ❑ Physics is difficult subject.
- ❑ They started late in afternoon.
- ❑ At top of banyan tree, there lived eagle.
- ❑ He likes to picturise himself as original artist.
- ❑ April is fourth month of year.
- ❑ Clouds over hill are lovely today.
- ❑ May I have pleasure of your company?
- ❑ Time makes worst of enemies friends.

1. Form as many sentences as you can from the table below and underline the articles.

There is	a boy	in this college.
There was	a girl	in the school.
There will be	an umbrella	on the platform.
Here is not	an apple	in the market.
Here was not	an old man	in that street.
Here will not be	a lame man	near the hall.

Note: The first three sentences are with **'There'**, *and the second three sentences are with,* **'Here'**. *All the three tenses,* **Present, Past and Future** *have been indicated in the formed sentences.*

2. Go through the table carefully and form as many sentences as possible with the help of the articles, 'a' and 'the'. Also underline the articles.

This picture		damaged	in an accident.
Her leg		shown	in the exhibition.
A new car	is	forgotten	by him.
A diner set	was	praised	outside the hall.
The fort		hit hard	in the market.
A necklace		examined	Near the Highway.

Note: All the sentences formed from the above table are both in **Present** *and* **Past Tenses** *and have both the articles,* **'a'** *and* **'the'**.

1. Complete the following sentences by filling in the blanks with 'a/an' or some:

Example: I ought to do _____ housework.

Answer: I ought to do some housework.

Nitin is here for two nights, and he is looking for _____ accommodation.

I can't fit this book into ___ bag.

He is doing _____ research on radioactivity.

We are just about to set off on _____ long journey.

The people who camped in the field have left---- rubbish.

This isn't right. Look, you've made_____ mistake.

The scientists are doing _____ interesting experiment.

You need _____ luck to win at this game.

English Grammar Workbook

My room is quite empty. We need ___ furniture.

I have been working on my essay. I think I've made____ progress.

You pay extra for the taxi if you have got____ luggage.

The second-hand shop had ____ table.

Note: All the sentences formed from the above table will be both in Present and Past Tenses with the determiners/articles, 'a' 'an' and 'the' and also underline these words in the sentences. However, all the sentences contain 'give' and 'gave' in them. So, their formation will be different.

Determiners

We use a number of words before common nouns (or adjective common noun) which we call determiners because they affect (or 'determine') the meaning of the noun. Determiners make it clear for example which particular thing(s) we are referring to or how much of a substance we are talking about. Singular countable nouns must normally have a determiner before them.

1. **Determiners which classify or identify**
   - ❑ Indefinite article   I bought a new pen yesterday
   - ❑ Definite article   The book I am reading is expensive
   - ❑ Demonstratives   I bought this/that table yesterday
   - ❑ Possessives   do you like my new car?

2. **Determiners which indicate quantity**
   - ❑ Numbers   I bought two new dresses yesterday.
   - ❑ Quantifiers   I didn't buy many apples today.

There wasn't much sugar in the house.

Determiners compared with pronouns

Determiners are always followed by a noun, words such as some and this followed by a noun function as determiners. When they stand on their own they function as pronouns:

I want some water (some+noun, functioning as determiner)

        I want this   I want some

Important Determiners

Articles: a, an, the

Demonstratives: this, these, that, those

Possessives: my, our, your, his, her, its, their

Some other determiners: some, any, much, many, many a, each every, few, a few, the few, little, the little, a little either, neither, all, whole, less, fewer

1. Some, any
   Some, when used with nouns to represent things that can be counted means a few or a small number. When used with a singular noun to represent something that cannot be counted 'some' means a little or a small quantity. Some is generally used in affirmative

sentences as:

I have bought some shirts.

Some men are born great.

Any expresses a small number with countable nouns and a small quantity with singular uncountable nouns. Any is used in this sense in questions and negative sentences:

Are there any files on my table?

Is there any tea in the kettle?

2. Much, many

Many mean a great number. Much means a large quantity. Many is used with countable nouns. Much is used with uncountable nouns; as,

Many people went to see the film.

I do not have many books.

3. Less, fewer

Less denotes quantity; as,

Please put less sugar in my coffee.

He had less money in his pocket.

Fewer denotes number; as,

There are fewer boys in this section than in that section.

No fewer than twenty girls were absent today.

4. All, whole

All denotes number as well as quantity; as,

He ate up all the sweets.

All men are mortal.

Whole and the whole denote quantity only; as

We have written the whole page.

The whole of the shop is on fire.

5. Each, every

Each refers to one of two or more things or persons, the emphasis being on the individual whole of a group of more than two taken individually.

Each girl will get a prize.

Each student was given a book.

6. Either, neither

Either means one of the two or both, as,

There are trees, on either side of the road.

You can go by either road.

Neither means not either or none of the two; as,

Neither side is winning.

She took neither side.

7. Few, a few, the few

'Few' means hardly any. It has a negative meaning:

Few men reach the age of a hundred years.

Few people are free from faults.
A few means a small number. It has a positive meaning:
He was asked to say a few words.
The few means not many, but all of them.
He lost the few friends he had.
The few clothes the tailor had were irreparable.

8. Little, a little, the little
Little means hardly any.
There is little hope of the patient's recovery.
There is little sugar left in the pot.
A little means some, though not much.
He has still a little money left in the bank.
A little knowledge is a dangerous thing.
The little means not much, but the whole of it:
I gave to the beggar the little money I had.

1. **Fill in the blanks with some, any, each, every, either, neither:**
   - ❑ ____ side has won.
   - ❑ ____ day has its problems.
   - ❑ It rained ____ day during the holidays.
   - ❑ We have ____ money.
   - ❑ We do not have ____ rice.
   - ❑ You may have ____ of the three books.
   - ❑ ____ players did his best.
   - ❑ He may take ____ side.
   - ❑ Will you bring me ____ honey?
   - ❑ ____ man must do his duty.

2. **Fill in the blanks with many, much, all, whole, the whole:**
   - ❑ ____ students attended the class.
   - ❑ She had ____ wealth.
   - ❑ The boxer ate the ____ loaf.
   - ❑ ____ are not lovers of nature.
   - ❑ We received ____ help from our neighbours.
   - ❑ The ____ family was plunged in grief.
   - ❑ ____ men are mortal.
   - ❑ ____ a boy was present today.
   - ❑ Tagore has written ____ books.
   - ❑ I ate a ____ pineapple.

1. **Form as many sentences as you can from the table below and identify by underlining the determiners.**

I		bright eyes.
You	have /have not	steady steps.
They	(haven't)	healthy cows.
Some singers		small houses.
Five actors		new bicycles.
A few teachers		adequate sugar.
Ten workers		big gardens.
Most of the farmers		sweet voice.
Some other men		mobile phones.
A few women		mango trees.
Young nurses		many relatives.
		grown up children

Note: You can frame both Positive and Negative sentences. However, all the sentences formed will be in Present Tense.

2. **Form as many sentences as you can from the table below and identify by underlining the determiners.**

I		bright eyes.
You	had/had not	steady steps.
They	(hadn't)	healthy cows.
Some dancers		small houses.
Five actors		new bicycles.
A few teachers		adequate sugar.
Ten labourers		big gardens.
Most of the farmers		sweet voice.
Some other men		mobile phones.
A few women		mango trees.
Young nurses		many relatives.
		grown up children

Note: You can frame both Positive and Negative sentences. However, all the sentences formed will be in Present Tense.

5. Form as many sentences as you can from the table below with the determiners, 'a few' and 'many'.

		match sticks in the match boxes.
There are	a few	books on the book shelf.
Are there	many	flowers in my garden.
There are not		flowering plants in my area.
		leaves on trees during winter.
		bags in the store.

Note: First complete all the sentences that you can make with **'a few'** *and then with* **'many'***, but the maximum number of sentences which you can form will be 36. The sentences formed with* **'Are there'** *will end with* **Question Marks** *(?).*

⸎⸎⸎

Chapter 5

Adjectives

Exercises

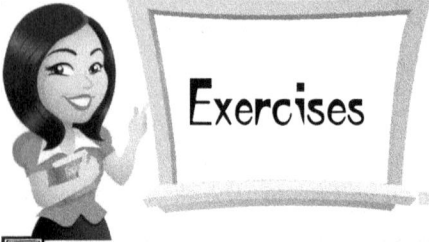

1. **Go through the table carefully and make as many sentences as you can. Also underline all the adjectives in the following sentences.**

			authentic flags.
These	are		street dogs.
Those	were		modern houses.
			pet birds.
			rough copies.
			intelligent boys.
			house plants.
			rainy coats.
			weather charts.
			race horses.
			steel chairs.
			regular beggars.
			green trees.
			old pants.
			new maps.
			Indian cows.
			mild animals.
			text books.
			working girls.
			new benches.
			half shirts.
			right keys.
			table fans.
			cheap mobiles.
			costly computers.

English Grammar Workbook

*Note: For Example: These are **authentic** flags.*

*These are **street** dogs.*

Kinds of Adjectives

Adjectives may be divided into the following classes:

1. **Adjectives of Quality answer the question: of what kind? They show the kind of quality of a person or thing; as,**
   - ❏ He is a *clever* boy.
   - ❏ *Indian* goods are sold abroad.
   - ❏ Adjectives formed from proper nouns (e.g., *Indian* goods, *French* perfumes, *English* language, etc.) are sometimes called Proper
   - ❏ Adjectives. They are generally classed with adjectives of Quality.

2. **Adjectives of Quantity**
   Adjectives of quantity answer the question, how much? They show how much of a thing is meant; as,
   - ❏ He ate *some* bread.
   - ❏ We have had *enough* exercise.

3. **Adjectives of Number answer the question, how many, or in what order. They show how many persons or things are meant, or in what order a person or thing stands; as,**
   Take *some* ripe bananas.

   Few boys want to take risks.

4. **Demonstrative Adjectives answer the question, 'which'? They point out which person or thing is meant; as,**
   - ❏ Those girls must be rewarded.
   - ❏ This boy is brave.
   1. Interrogative Adjectives
   - ❏ Interrogative adjectives are used with nouns to ask question; as,
   - ❏ Whose shirt is this?
   - ❏ Which road leads to the town?

   2. Emphasising Adjectives
   - ❏ Emphasizing adjectives are own and very; as,
   - ❏ I saw it with my own eyes.
   - ❏ This is the very man who killed the tiger.
   3. Exclamatory Adjectives
   - ❏ What is sometimes used as an exclamatory adjective; as,
   - ❏ What an idea! What luck!
   - ❏ What a piece of work man is!

Adjectives Used as Nouns

Adjectives are sometimes used as nouns: as,

1. **Certain adjectives,** *preceded by the,* **can be used as nouns in the plural sense. They denote a class of persons:**
    Blessed are the meek
    The rich do not care for the poor.

2. **Some adjectives, preceded by the, denote some abstract quality:**
    The future is unknown to us.
    He admires the good.

3. **Some adjectives actually become nouns and can be used both in the singular and in the plural:**
    ❏ Junior, juniors; senior, seniors; Italian, Italians; superior, superiors; elder, elders; mortals; inferior, inferiors; Indian, Indians, etc.

4. **In certain phrases and idioms, the adjectives are used as nouns:**
    ❏ I shall see you before long.

🅑

1. **Form as many sentences as you can and underline the adjectives. Also specify the kind of adjective in each case.**

			very hot day?	
			wintery night?	
Is	it	not a/the	Sunday afternoon?	?
was	that		month of April?	
			a sunny day?	
			cloudy sky?	
			foggy weather?	
			a dense forest?	
			a beautiful garden?	
			a cool evening?	
			a delicious dish?	
			a rough way?	
			a mammoth gathering?	
			the public opinion?	
			the general rule?	

Note: All the sentences formed from the above table end with **Question Marks** *and are* **Negative Sentences**.

2. **Form as many sentences as you can from the table given below, then identify and underline the adjectives. Also specify the kind of adjective in each case.**

		five flags.
There		big houses.
	are	small birds.
	were	plenty of boys.
		tall plants.
		innumerable coats.
		black horses.
		uncomfortable chairs.
		huge trees.
		only blue pants.
		two world maps.
		few old cows.
		some religious books.
		a whole lot of benches.
		bright shirts.
		no keys here.

Note: All the sentences formed from the above table are **plural** *in number and are both in* **Present** *and* **Past Tenses**.

3. **Form as many sentences as you can from the table below, then underline the adjectives. Also specify the kind of adjective in each case.**

			authentic flags.
			street dogs.
These	are	not	modern houses.
Those	were		rough copies.
			intelligent boys.
			weather charts.
			race horses.
			wild animals.
			working girls.
			cheap mobiles.
			costly computers.

Note: All the sentences formed from the above table are **plural** *in number and are* **negative** *in character.*

4. **Form as many sentences as you can from the table below, then underline the adjectives. Also specify the kind of adjective in each case.**

		big eyes.
She	has	strong legs.
He	has not	a new bicycle.
Suman		a pot of sugar.
A singer		a kitchen garden.
An actor		a big house.
A teacher		long nose.
A worker		a computer.
A farmer		some fruit trees.
A potter		

Note: *All the sentences formed will have* **'Has'** *and* **'Has not'***, i.e., they are in* **singular number** *and are of both* **Positive** *and* **Negative** *character.*

5. **Form as many sentences as you can from the table below, then underline the adjectives. Also specify the kind of adjective in each case.**

		bright eyes.
I		healthy cows.
You	have	small houses.
They		new bicycles.
Ten actors		adequate sugar.
A few teachers		sweet voice.
Four workers		mango trees.
Most of the farmers		many relatives.
A few women		grown-up children.
Some nurses		

Note: *All the sentences formed will have* **'Have'** *and* **'Have not'***, i.e., they are in* **singular number** *and are of both* **Positive** *and* **Negative** *character.*

Chapter 6

Degrees of Comparison

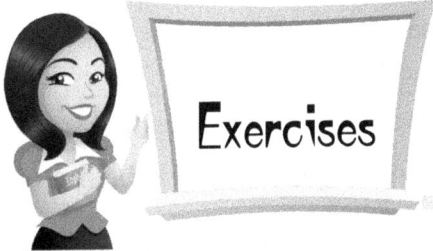

Exercises

A

1. **Change the degree of comparison without changing the meaning:**
   1. Australia is the largest island in the world.
   2. A wise enemy is better than a foolish friend.
   3. Hunger is the best sauce.
   4. Very few countries are as rich as America.
   5. No other man is as strong as Atul.
   6. Shakespeare is greater than any other English poet.
   7. No other exercise is as convenient as swimming.
   8. Hyderabad is not so cool as Bangalore.

2. **Fill in the blanks with 'elder', eldest, older or oldest:**
   1. He is the _____ man in our village.
   2. She is my ___ sister.
   3. He is the _____ of the two brothers.
   4. She is _____ than Seema.
   5. Rita is the ___ girls in the school.
   6. This is the ___ temple in Goa.
   7. She is _____ than my brother.
   8. Of the two brothers Aseem is the _____.

1. **Make as many sentences as you can with the words given in the table below and underline the degrees of comparison.**

This young man		Idle	
This boy		truthful	as that.
This girl	is as	wicked	
This merchant	is not as	popular	
This river	is not so	greedy	
This manager		famous	

Note: All the sentences formed above will be in the **Positive Degree of Comparison.**

2. **Make as many sentences as you can with the words given in the table below and underline the degrees of comparison.**

I saw	the tallest tree.
He saw	the most beautiful city.
She saw	the highest mountain.
They visited	the oldest person.
They live near	the longest field.
We are very close to	the largest stadium.
	the biggest market.

Note: All the sentences formed above will be in **Superlative Degree of Comparison** *and should have* **'the'** *before the Superlative Degree.*

3. **Make as many sentences as you can with the words given in the table below and underline the degrees of comparison. Also specify the type of the degree of comparison in each case.**

This leader			
This teacher		the greatest	of all.
This young man	is	the wisest	
This boy	was	the most worthy	
This rich man	will be	more popular	
This merchant		more learned	
This river		more honest	
This leader		more diligent	

Note: You can form as many sentences as you can but all the sentences will begin with **'This'** *and end with* **'of all'.**

English Grammar Workbook

4. **Comparisons: Make as many comparative sentences as you can with 'is more' and 'is less'.**

This young man This boy This girl This rich man This merchant This river This leader This manager	is more is less	idle truthful wicked popular greedy famous dangerous	than that.

Note: All the above sentences formed will start with **'this'** *and end with* **'that'**, *and the maximum number of sentences formed will be 147.*

5. **Comparisons: Make as many comparative sentences as you can with 'is more' and 'is less'.**

That young man That boy That girl That rich man That merchant That river That leader That manager	is more is less	idle truthful wicked popular greedy famous dangerous	than this.

Note: All the above sentences formed will start with 'this' and end with 'that'. For example: That young man is more idle than this. That boy is more idle than this, That girl is more idle than this, That man is more rich than this and so on...

⚜

Chapter 7

Verbs

Exercises

A

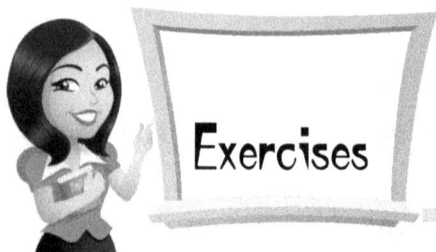

1. Underline the verbs in the following sentences.

1. He raised a difficult question.
2. She is good at assessing people.
3. We should de-emphasise the dangers of the situation.
4. I am returning the raincoat I borrowed.
5. The wine had been diluted.
6. I want to organize my photographs.
7. We discussed the situation.
8. May I test your bicycle?
9. You can collect the tickets at the box office.
10. Do you think they invented the whole story?

2. Underline the verbs in these sentences and specify the type in each case.

1. The mailman delivered the letter next door.
2. James calls his friends on the weekends.
3. The children played in the morning.
4. My mother usually makes tea in the morning.
5. The soldiers celebrated last week.
6. Andrea went to the beach last Sunday.
7. They stood in line for hours waiting for the doors to open.
8. He showed us his wedding album.
9. Tom forgot his homework at home.
10. The teacher just arrived.

1. Form as many sentences as you can and identify and underline the verbs.

		to write a story.
I	give/gave him advice	to play outdoor games.
We	give/gave her advice	to take medicine regularly.
He		to take sweets after meal.
She		to read good books.
They		to avoid overeating.
The teachers		to go to bed early.
The doctor		to walk fast.
		to munch the food.
		to draw portraits.

*Note: All the above sentences are both in **Present** and **Past Tense**.*

2. Form as many sentences as you can and identify and underline the verbs.

		Sanskrit.
I		Hindi.
We	taught him	English.
He	taught her	History.
She	gave lessons in	Science.
They		Hindi Grammar.
The teachers		Scriptures.
The doctor		Ethics.
		how to read.
		how to write.
		how to sing.

*Note: All the above sentences are in **Past Tense** only.*

3. **Form as many sentences as you can and identify and underline the verbs. Also write the type of the verb in each case.**

He	moves fast.
She	runs slow.
A man	plays well.
A boy	creates ideas.
Sohan	holds a map.
Nita	drinks juice on rare occasions.
	tells nice stories.
	works in a factory.
	carries a bag everyday.
	prefers a high stool.
	plays with mobile phones.

Note: Form all the sentences that you can with **one verb**, *then move to the* **next verb**. *In this way, make as many sentences as you can.*

4. **Given below is a table from which form as many sentences as you can and underline the verbs. Also specify its type in each case.**

I am	dividing the profit.
He is	learning something.
She is	walking slowly.
A boy is	forcing others.
A girl is	helping others.
The boy is	talking sweetly.
The girl is	sitting idle.
The hawker is	asking for action.
We are	paying the fare.
They are	collecting articles.
You are	throwing garbage.
The traders are	laughing loudly.
The workers are	working swiftly.

Note: All the verbs in the above sentences from the table end with **'ing'** *and are in* **Present Tense-** *denoting* **Present Continuous Tense**.

English Grammar Workbook

5. **Make as many sentences as you can from the table given below and underline the verbs specifying its type in each case.**

I was	dividing the profit.
He was	learning something.
She was	walking slowly.
A boy was	forcing others.
A girl was	helping others.
The boy was	talking sweetly.
The girl was	sitting idle.
The hawker was	asking for action.
We were	paying the fare.
They were	collecting articles.
You were	throwing garbage.
The traders were	laughing loudly.

Note: All the above formed sentences are in **Past Continuous Tense***, i.e., the work is being done in the past tense, but it's not complete and is still going on.*

6. **Form as many sentences as you can from the table below. Also underline the verb in each case.**

She	has	finished the work.
He		accepted the guilt.
The golfer		punished others.
The player		claimed the share.
The singer		visited the shrine.
The hawker		completed the task.
The shopkeeper		counted the flowers.

Note: All the above formed sentences have verbs as **'has'** *and ending with* **'ed'***.*

7. **Form as many sentences as you can from the table below. Also underline the verb in each case.**

I	have/have not or haven't	finished the work.
We		accepted the guilt.
You		punished others.
They		claimed the share.
The players		visited the shrine.
The singers		completed the task.
The shopkeepers		counted the flowers.

Note: All the above formed sentences have helping verbs as **'have'** *or* **'have not'** **(haven't)** *and the main verbs ending with* **'ed'**. *This is also called as the* **Present Perfect Tense**.

8. **Form as many sentences as you can from the table below. Also underline the verb specifying its type in each case.**

I	had/had not or hadn't	finished the work.
We		accepted the guilt.
You		punished others.
They		claimed the share.
The players		visited the shrine.
The singers		completed the task.
The shopkeepers		counted the flowers.

Note: All the above formed sentences have verbs as **'had'** *or* **had not (hadn't)** *as the helping verbs and the main verbs ending with* **'ed'**. *This is also called as the* **Past Perfect Tense**.

Chapter 8

Agreement of the Verb with The Subject

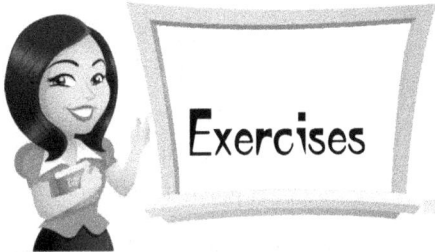

Exercises

A

1. Fill in the blanks with the correct forms of the verbs given in brackets:

1. The quality of pens _____ good (is/are).
2. A white and a black cow _____ grazing in the field (is/are).
3. Namrata, as well as her friends _____ present(is/are).
4. Each of these minerals _____found in India. (is/are).
5. The chief with all his men _____killed (was/were).
6. The committee _____ elected its president. (has/have)
7. He is one of the greatest leaders that _____ ever lived (has/have)
8. If your braces_____ loose, your trousers_____ down (is/are, comes/come).
9. The dancer and singer _____ arrived (has/have).
10. The Arabian Nights _____ an interesting book. (is/arc).

2. Supply a verb in agreement with the subject in each of the following sentences:

1. What_____ the news? My glasses_____ lost and I cannot read.
2. The voice of the singers _____ pleasant.
3. Many an attempt _____ been made to climb Mount Everest.
4. The shop, with all its contents, _____ insured.
5. Which of those books _____ yours?
6. Ten thousand rupees _____ a big sum.
7. Neither of my uncles _____ any children.
8. This is the only one of her poems that _____ worth reading.
9. Either Manisha or I _____ to blame.
10. The great poet and singer_____ dead.

1. **Make as many sentences as you can from the table below and identify and underline the verb in agreement with the subject in each case.**

			A good teacher.
			a famous painter.
Hema's	brother	is	an active politician
Rajesh's	sister	was	a dull worker.
His	mother	will be	a rich lawyer.
My	father		a popular doctor.
Her	uncle		a hard worker.
Our	aunt		a smooth runner.
Their	nephew		a perfect magician.
Your			a pop singer.
			a great artist.
			very happy.
			very tired.
			very serious.
			very angry.
			seriously ill.
			extremely happy.

Note: All the sentences formed will be in **Present, Past** *and* **Future Tense**.

2. **Form as many sentences as you can from the table below and identify and underline the verb in agreement with the subject in each case.**

There is	a boy	in this college.
There was	a girl	in the school.
There will be	a player	on the platform.
There is not	a doctor	in the market.
There was not	a crowd	in that street.
There will not be	a lame man	near the hall.

Note: All the sentences begin with **'There'**, *and are in* **Present**, **Past** *and* **Future Tense**. *Some are* **Positive** *and some are* **Negative** *sentences.*

3. **Form as many sentences as you can from the table below and identify by underlining the verb in agreement with the subject in each case.**

		big eyes.
She	has	strong legs.
He	has not (hasn't)	shapely arms.
Shashi		a red cow.
They		a black horse.
A singer		a new bicycle.
An actor		a pot of sugar.
A teacher		a kitchen garden.
A worker		a big house.
A farmer		a computer.
A potter		some fruit trees.

Note: All the sentences are in the **Present Tense** *with* '**Has**' *and in* **singular** *number. Some are* **Positive** *and some are* **Negative** *sentences.*

4. **Form as many sentences as you can from the table below and identify by underlining the verb in agreement with the subject in each case.**

I		bright eyes.
You	have	steady steps.
They		healthy cows.
Some singers	have not (haven't)	small houses.
Five actors		new bicycles.
A few teachers		adequate sugar.
Ten workers		big gardens.
Most of the farmers		sweet voice.
Some other men		mobile phones.
A few women		mango trees.
Young nurses		many relatives.
		grown up children.

Note: All the sentences have verbs in the **Present Tense** *with* '**Have**' *and are in* **plural** *number. However, some are* **Positive** *and some are* **Negative** *sentences.*

5. Make as many sentences as you can from the table below and identify by underlining the verb in agreement with the subject in each case.

She		big eyes.
He	had	strong legs.
Rekha	had not (hadn't)	shapely arms.
They		a red cow.
A singer		a black horse.
An actor		a new bicycle.
A teacher		a pot of sugar.
A worker		a kitchen garden.
A farmer		a big house.
A potter		a computer.
		some fruit trees.

Note: All the sentences have verbs in the Past Tense with **'Had'** *and* **Had not** *or* **Hadn't** *, i.e., some sentences are* **Positive** *and some are* **Negative** *Sentences.*

Chapter-9

Gerunds

Exercises

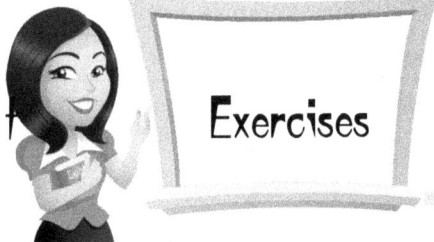

1. Put the verbs in brackets into the gerund form:

1. Sunita does not enjoy (go) to the dentist.
2. I hate (borrow) money.
3. Would you mind (write) your address on the form?
4. Stop (argue) and start (think).
5. He is thinking of (make) his will.
6. Is there anything there worth (buy)?
7. It's no use (cry) over spilt milk.
8. She is looking forward to (read) your article.
9. I remember (read) a review of that film.
10. He finished (speak) and left the hall.

1. Form as many sentences as you can from the table below and identify and underline the gerunds.

Please stop	talking.
He enjoys	playing tennis.
I remember	doing it.
Please excuse	me for being so late.
Do you mind	staying a little longer?
Do you mind	my for staying a little longer?
She could not	laughing.
He keeps on	coming here.
They went on	talking.
Has it left off	raining yet.

Note: Combine each of the first part with each of the second part to frame separate sentences.

Subject + Verb	Gerund etc
He began	talking./ to talk.
He likes	swimming./ to swim.
I prefer	staying indoors./ to stay indoors.
I hate	refusing every time./ to refuse every time.
He started	packing books./ to pack his books.

Note: Form as many sentences as you can but the maximum number of sentences that you can form with the above gerunds will be: 25 + 25=50

2. Subject + Verb + Gerund

Subject + Verb + Gerund, etc.

Subject + Verb	Gerund
Please stop	talking.
He enjoys	playing tennis.
I remember	doing it.
Please excuse	me being so late.
Do you mind	staying a little longer?
Do you mind	my staying a little longer?
She could not	laughing.
He keeps on	coming here.
They went on	talking.
Has it left off	raining yet.

Note: Form as many sentences as you can with the help of the above Gerunds but the maximum number of sentences that you will get=100.

3. Subject + Verb + Gerund, etc.

Combine each of the first part with each of the second part to frame separate sentences.

Subject + Verb	Gerund etc
He began	talking./ to talk.
He likes	swimming./ to swim.
I prefer	staying indoors./ to stay indoors.
I hate	refusing every time./ to refuse every time.
He started	packing books./ to pack his books.

Note: Form as many sentences as you can with the help of the above Gerunds, etc., but the maximum number of sentences that you will get=25+25=50

4. Combine each of the first part with each of the second part, to frame separate sentences.

Subject + Verb	Gerund etc (Passive Infinite)
It needs	elaborating. / to be elaborated.
Your work needs	correcting. / to be corrected.
That needs	explaining. / to be explained.
He needs	refreshing. / to be refreshed.
Number of sentences	16 + 16

Note: *Form as many sentences as you can with the help of the above Gerunds, etc., but the maximum number of sentences that you will get=16+16=32. Here the Gerunds, etc., are being used as* **Passive Infinitives**.

⚜️

Chapter-10

Modal Auxiliary Verbs or Modals

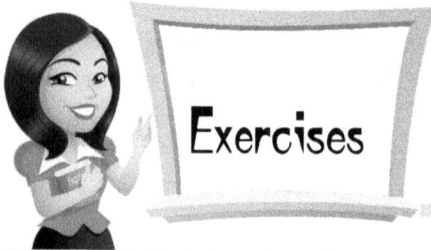

Exercises

1. Fill in the blanks with 'shall, will, should or would'.

1. We _____ speak the truth.
2. A dog _____ always remains faithful to his master.
3. Amit said that he _____ not talk to her any more.
4. A self-respecting man_____ rather die than tell lies.
5. As you sow, so _____ you reap.
6. You _____ be punished if you don't do the work.
7. The old man is walking with care lest he _____ stumble.
8. If I were you, I _____ not do it.
9. If today is Saturday, tomorrow _____ be Sunday.

2. Fill in the blanks with 'need, used to, ought to dare or must'.

1. He _____ call on me today.
2. Pupil's _____respect their teachers.
3. How _____ you enter my house?
4. One _____ obey the traffic rules.
5. A judge ___- be honest.
6. He ____- to do this heavy work.
7. They ___-- go out on Sundays.
8. _____ I remind you of your promise?
9. It ___ be done with great care.
10. He _____ not write to his grandfather.

3. **Fill in the blanks with 'must, needn't, can, could, may, might, ought to, and should'.**

   1. _____ my friend live long!

   2. You _____ have been more careful.

   3. Criminals___ be punished.

   4. She _____ speak French when she was seven years old.

   5. It _____ happen, but I don't think it will.

   6. A cook _____ prepare the food with care.

   7. We _____ always obey our superiors.

   8. Visitors_____ not go beyond this limit.

   9. I _____ help you if I have time.

   10. We _____ hear people talking in the hall.

B

1. **Make as many sentences as you can with the words given in the table below and identify the modals by underlining them.**

I shall	run	for an hour
We shall	play	for a prize.
They shall	go	for health.
He will	sing	for growth.
She will	stay	for a position
The teacher will	sleep	for a medal.
The tutor will	drink	in the field.
The passenger will	drive	in dress.
The player will	call	in the school.
The girls will	cry	
The clerks will		

Note: All the sentences formed above will be in **Simple Future Tense or Future Indefinite Tense**, *and you can make as many as 990 sentences.*

2. **Make as many sentences as you can with the words given in the table below and identify the modals by underlining them.**

I shall		encouraging others.
We shall	be	discouraging others.
They shall		blaming others.
He will		praising others.
She will		talking in vain.
The teacher will		delivering a lecturer.
The tutor will		carrying the bag.

The passenger will		typing a letter.
The player will		starting the computer.
The girls will		watching the match.
The clerks will		buying a ticket.

Note: *All the sentences formed above will be in* **Future Imperfect Tense** *or* **Future Continuous Tense**, *and you can make as many as 121 sentences.*

❧❧❧

Adverbs

Exercises

A

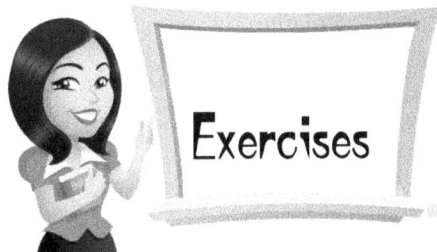

1. **Fill in the blanks with the suitable words:**
   - ❑ He spoke loud _____ to be heard. (much, enough).
   - ❑ It is _____ late, but not _____ late to catch the train. (too, very)
   - ❑ She waited for us _____ impatiently. (very, much)
   - ❑ Fruit is _____ cheap today, but is _____ dear for me to buy any. (too, very)
   - ❑ This magazine is _____ heavy, but that one is _____ light. (fairly, rather)
   - ❑ This news is _____ good to be true (very, too)
   - ❑ It is _____ hot to go outside. (very, much)
   - ❑ Our school closed a fortnight _____ (since, ago)
   - ❑ She has been absent from school _____ last Monday. (since, ago)
   - ❑ The patient is _____ - better today. (too, much)

2. **Insert the words in the brackets in suitable places:**
   - ❑ We lost the match. (nearly)
   - ❑ He makes a mistake. (rarely)
   - ❑ He did well in the examination. (fairly)
   - ❑ The pupils have completed the class work. (almost)
   - ❑ I am late for my lectures. (often)
   - ❑ Does he make mistakes? (generally)
   - ❑ I was able to hear what they said. (hardly)
   - ❑ He has travelled by train. (never)
   - ❑ We deceive ourselves. (sometimes)
   - ❑ I know her well. (quite)

1. **Form as many sentences as you can from the table given below and underline the adverbs. Also specify its kind in each case.**

He	does/does not(doesn't)	move fast.
She		run slowly.
It		play well.
A man		drinks juice rarely.
A boy		tell interesting stories daily.
The man		work hard in a factory.
The boy		carry a bag every day.
Sohan		play with mobile phones usually.
Neeta		

Note: Each of the sentences formed from the above table have **helping verbs, 'does'** *or* **does not (doesn't)** *followed by the main verb and an adverb in each case. However, all the sentences will be in* **Present Tense**.

2. **Form as many sentences as you can from the table given below and underline the adverbs. Also specify its kind in each case.**

He	did/did not	move fast.
She	(didn't)	run slowly.
It		play well.
A man		drinks juice rarely.
A boy		tell interesting stories daily.
The man		work hard in a factory.
The boy		carry a bag every day.
Sohan		play with mobile phones smartly.
Neeta		

Note: Each of the sentences formed from the above table will have **helping verbs, 'did'** *or* **did not (didn't)** *followed by the main verb and an adverb in each case. However, all the sentences formed will be in* **Past Tense**.

3. **Form as many sentences as you can from the table given below and underline the adverbs. Also specify its kind in each case.**

He	is/are	singing melodiously
She		writing letters continuously.
We		calling someone loudly.

They		going for a walk regularly.
A teacher		coming towards the temple quickly.
The manager		teaching some people occasionally.
A devotee		cleaning the table regularly.
		arranging papers neatly.

*Note: Each of the sentences formed from the above table will have a **helping verb is/are**, as the case may be followed by the main verb and then the adverb. However, all the sentences will be in Present Continuous Tense, i.e., expressing the work is not complete, but is going on.*

4. **Form as many sentences as you can from the table given below and underline the adverbs. Also specify its kind in each case.**

	is/are	
He		singing melodiously
She		writing letters continuously.
We		calling someone loudly.
They		going for a walk regularly.
A teacher		coming towards the temple quickly.
The manager		teaching some people occasionally.
A devotee		cleaning the table regularly.
		arranging papers neatly.

*Note: Each of the sentences formed from the above table will have a **helping verb was/were**, as the case may be followed by the main verb and then the adverb. However, all the sentences will be in **Past Continuous Tense**, i.e., indicating that the work was not complete, but was going on.*

Chapter-12

Prepositions

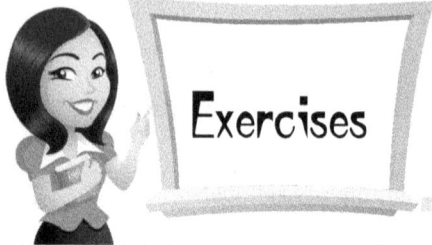

Exercises

1. Choose a suitable preposition from the options given in each bracket.

❑ The children sat (on/upon) the ground.

❑ One should live (in/within) one's means.

❑ We must trust (in/on) our close friends.

❑ The train is (after/behind) time.

❑ Three thieves quarreled (between/among) themselves.

❑ He arrived (by/with) all his belongings.

❑ She was (in/at) Kolkata last night.

❑ She has been ill (since/for) last night.

❑ We will return (in/on an hour.

❑ We returned from the picnic (after/since) three days.

1. Subject + Verb + Direct Object + Preposition + Prepositional Object

Subject + Verb		Preposition	
I gave	the money	to	my friend.
They told	the news	to	everybody they met.
We showed	the pictures	to	our teachers.
I do not lend	my books	to	anybody.
He offered	once	to	me.
I owe	30 rupees	to	my tailor.
Throw	that box	to	me.
Bring	that book	to	me.

English Grammar Workbook

Note: Combine the first part with the second part and use the preposition,' to' to form eight different types of sentences.

2. Subject + Verb+ Direct Object + Preposition + Prepositional Object

Subject + Verb	Direct Object	Preposition	Prepositional object
He bought	a necklace	for	the bride.
He gifted	a gold watch	to	his wife.
Please give	some	for	me.
They left	a message	for	the commander.
She made	a new dress	for	herself.
Have you left	any	for	your sister.
Please get	two tickets	for	me.
They selected	a bride	for	their son.

Note: Form as many sentences as you can using appropriate prepositions from the above table and the maximum number of sentences that you can get will be = 8

3. Subject + Verb+ Direct Object + Preposition + Prepositional Object

Subject + Verb	Direct Object	Preposition	Prepositional Object
Thank	You	for	your kind help.
Ask	him	for	a few more.
Compare	this	with	that flag.
They punished	him	for	being very late.
Congratulate	him	on	his grand success.
Do not throw	the stone	at	the poor donkey.
What prevented	you	from	joining the post?
Add	this	to	what you have.
I explained	my difficulty	to	the manager.
Protect	us	from	the terrorists.

Note: Form as many sentences as you can using appropriate prepositions from the above table and the maximum number of sentences that you can get will be =10

4. Form as many sentences as you can and identify by underlining the prepositions.

		is calling me.
	under the tree,	is playing a game.
The girl,	at the window,	is holding a book.
The boy,	in the classroom,	is blowing a whistle.
The teacher,	on the road,	is writing a letter.
The man,		is eating a fruit.
The woman,		is driving a car.
		is asking for help.

Note: You can make as many sentences as you can, but all the sentences formed will be in Present Continuous Tense or Present Imperfect Tense indicating that the work is under process and not complete.

5. Form as many sentences as you can and identify by underlining the prepositions.

		is not calling me.
	above the tree,	is not playing a game.
The girl,	behind the window,	is not holding a book.
The boy,	near the classroom,	is not blowing a whistle.
The teacher,	across the road,	is not writing a letter.
The man,		is not eating a fruit.
The woman,		is not driving a car.
		is not asking for help.

*Note: You can make as many sentences as you can, but all the sentences formed will be Negative in nature and in **Present Continuous** or **Present Imperfect Tense**.*

6. Form as many sentences that you can form and underline the prepositions.

		book		
There is	a	pen	at	the table.
There was		pencil	on	the box.
There will be		chalk	near	the bag.
		lamp	by	my copy.
		knife	away from	that radio.
		slate	close to	the computer.
		ring	across	his diary.
		key	under	

Note: The maximum number of sentences that you can form will be 405. Underline all the prepositions.

⚜⚜

Chapter-13

Conjunctions

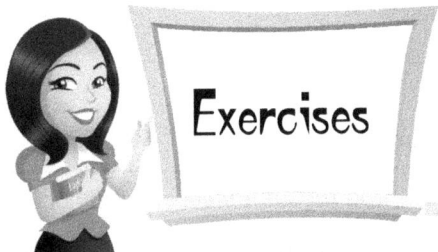

Exercises

1. Fill in the blanks with appropriate conjunctions:

- ❑ She was ___ill___ she could not study.
- ❑ Strike ____ the iron is hot.
- ❑ ____ she is poor,___ she is honest.
- ❑ ____ he tells the truth, he will be spared.
- ❑ I brought it ____ I needed it.
- ❑ Many strange things have happened___ they came here.
- ❑ Take heed ____ you fall.
- ❑ Please write____ she dictates.
- ❑ Make hay___ the sun shines.
- ❑ Rita is pretty ____ not proud.

2. Join each pair of sentences into one by using a suitable conjunction: One has been done for you.

- ❑ *Example: Rita has no time to answer your call as she is late.*
- ❑ We will go for an outing. We will do so if the weather is fine.
- ❑ We had better get ready now. We may not have time to reach the airport.
- ❑ Mr. Harry has been sick. He has been so since coming back from Japan.
- ❑ Do not start the rehearsal yet. The chairman has not arrived.
- ❑ The debating teams were very happy. Both were declared joint-champions.
- ❑ The players gave their best. They still did not win the match.
- ❑ The boys were unhappy with their results. The girls were also unhappy with theirs.

❑   Let us be more serious in our revision. We may not perform as well as we want.

B

1. Form as many sentences as you can and identify by underlining the conjunctions.

Is Was	the dog	white or black	?
	the cat	big or small	
	the horse	red or gray	
	the bag	mine or yours	
	the car	cheap or costly	
	the scooter	ugly or attractive	
	mobile phone	simple or majestic	

Note: All the sentences formed will end in Question Marks and the total number of sentences formed will be equal to 98.

2. Identify and underline the conjunctions in the sentences given below.

❑   The thief ran away when he saw the guard.

❑   Aunt will get angry if you do not come soon.

❑   He won the race even though he participated unwillingly.

❑   The sky turned cloudy and it began to rain.

❑   The boy became sad when the girl started crying.

❑   The girl looks innocent even though she is very clever.

❑   She continued to study though she had finished her course.

❑   The old man did not walk because he was very weak.

❑   We will attend the party even if you do not return back in time.

❑   I like to go to the countryside because it is free from pollution.

✻✻✻

Chapter-14

Interjection

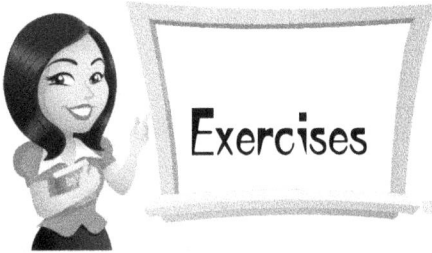

Exercises

1. **Fill in the blanks with the correct Interjections in the sentences given below.**
   - ❑ _____, that feels good!
   - ❑ _____, she's dead now!
   - ❑ _____! Does it hurt ?
   - ❑ _____! What do you think of that ?
   - ❑ _____! Didn't you know Lima is the capital of Peru.
   - ❑ _____ John, How are you today ?
   - ❑ _____ , I'm not so sure.
   - ❑ _____! 85 divided by 5 is17.
   - ❑ _____, Shall we go ?
   - ❑ _____! That hurts !

2. **Identify and underline the interjections in the sentences listed below.**
   - ❑ Hey! You left me behind.
   - ❑ Ouch! That soup is hot.
   - ❑ Oops! The plate broke
   - ❑ Well, I guess Ill go.
   - ❑ Hurray! We won the game.
   - ❑ Wow! John hit the ball far.
   - ❑ Hurry! I saw something scary in the cave.
   - ❑ Alas! I cannot go with you.
   - ❑ Shh! I heard something.
   - ❑ Ah, I see what you mean.

3. **Identify and underline the interjections in the sentences listed below.**
   - ❑ Hush! Don't disturb the class.
   - ❑ Alas! My friend has met with an accident.
   - ❑ Hurrah! They have won the match.
   - ❑ Bravo! We are going to Goa next week.
   - ❑ Ah! He is dead.
   - ❑ May he survive this crisis!
   - ❑ What a nice day!
   - ❑ How stupid of you to behave like this!
   - ❑ What a fool you are!
   - ❑ Oh! I'm having a terrible pain in stomach.

❖❖❖

Chapter-15

Tenses and their Uses

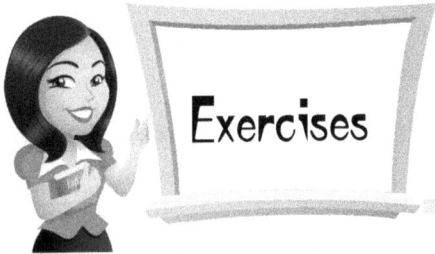

Exercises

1. **Fill in the blanks using the simple present or the present continuous tense of the words given in brackets:**
   - ❑ Where_____ you_____ now?" "I ___ to the theatre."(go)
   - ❑ Mr. Gupta ____ (teach) us English every day. He is absent: so Mr. Kumar ____ (take) our class just now.
   - ❑ The sun ___ (rises) in the east.
   - ❑ She generally ____ a red skirt but today she ____ a green one. (wear)
   - ❑ I ____ (drink) at least six glasses of water every morning.

2. **Use the past continuous tense in the following sentences:**
   - ❑ It _____ heavily all night. (rain)
   - ❑ ____ Football yesterday? (they play)
   - ❑ I _____, so I missed what he said. (not listen)
   - ❑ I ____ whether you could lend me your car. (wonder)
   - ❑ He ____ all weekend. (garden)
   - ❑ ____ when he left? (you still work)
   - ❑ ____ when she came to you? (you read)
   - ❑ I lived in Patna, when you _____ in Delhi? (live)
   - ❑ When he was young, he _____ football. (always play)

3. **Fill in the blanks with suitable forms of verbs given in brackets.**
   - ❑ The school bus ____ at school now. It ____ there since mid-day. (wait)
   - ❑ Amit always ___ (come) to school on time.

- ❑ She normally ____ very well but today she _____ very badly. (play)
- ❑ The sun ___ (shine) brightly when he got up this morning.
- ❑ I always ____ my raincoat in case it rains. I ____ my raincoat because it is likely to rain. (carry)
- ❑ He realized that he ____ (take) the wrong road.
- ❑ The telephone bell ___ (ring). It sometimes ____ fifty times a day. (ring).
- ❑ Vandana said that she ____ (see) that movie before.
- ❑ My brother ____ to the court every day. He ____ there now.(drive)
- ❑ The old man ____ (fall) as he (cross) the street.

1. Form as many sentences as you can and identify the Tense of the Verb in each case.

He	moves fast.
She/ It	runs slow.
A man	plays well.
A woman	creates ideas.
A boy	holds a map.
A girl	drinks juice on rare occasions.
Sohan	tells nice stories.
Nita	works in a factory.
	carries a bag everyday.
	prefers a high stool.
	plays with mobile phones.

Note: *You can form as many sentences as you can but the* **Noun/Pronoun** *in the* **first person** *is in* **singular number** *in all the sentences.*

2. Form as many sentences as you can and identify the Tense of the Verb in each case.

I	work hard.
We	lead a tough life.
They	show great skill.
Workers	perform well.
Officers	help the society.
Players	live for others.
Writers	sense the danger in time.
Students	take safety measures.

Farmers Drivers	come in time. sit for hours.

Note: Except for the first sentence, in all the other sentences, the **Noun/Pronoun** *in the* **first person** *is* **plural** *in number.*

3. Form as many sentences as you can and identify the Tense of the Verb in each case.

I am	dividing the profit.
He is	learning something.
She is	walking slowly.
A boy is	forcing others.
A girl is	helping others.
The hawker is	talking sweetly.
We are	sitting idle.
They are	asking for action.
Traders are	paying the fare.
Workers are	collecting articles.
Peons are	throwing garbage.

Note: Make as many sentences as you can and the maximum number of sentences you will get is 121.

4. Form as many sentences as you can and identify the Tense of the Verb in each case.

She	has	finished the work.
He		accomplished all.
The golfer		accepted the guilt.
The player		punished others.
The singer		claimed the share.
The hawker		visited the shrine.
The shopkeeper		completed the task.
		created some space.
		controlled the crowd.
		counted the flowers.
		shown the way.

Note: Make as many sentences as you can but the **Noun/Pronoun in the first person** *in all the sentences will be in* **singular number**.

5. Form as many sentences as you can and identify the Tense of the Verb in each case.

I	have	finished the work.
We		accomplished all.
Boys		accepted the guilt.
Girls		punished others.
His pupils		claimed the share.
My sons		grown up strong.
The salesmen		visited the shrine.
The representatives		completed the task.
The workers		controlled the crowd.
		counted the flowers.
		shown the way.

*Note: Make as many sentences as you can but the **Noun/Pronoun** in the **first person** in all the sentences will be in **plural number**.*

6. Form as many sentences as you can and identify the Tense of the Verb in each case.

He	has been	worrying since the last meal.
She		trying very hard for square meals.
It		looking into water.
A porter		working since morning.
A heron		visiting places.
A hermit		searching something in the soil.
A farmer		living on the least.
I	have been	facing dangers.
We		fighting for survival.
They		wasting time.
Birds		moving aimlessly.
Animals		doing nothing.
Insects		turning again and again.
Farmers		waiting for long.
Larks		Eating slowly.

Note: The maximum number of sentences that you can make will be 105+120=225.

English Grammar Workbook

7. Present Indefinite Interrogative

Do	I	work hard?
	we	lead a tough life?
	they	show great skill?
	workers	perform well?
	officers	help the society?
	players	live for others?
	writers	sense the danger in time?
	students	take safety measures?
	farmers	come in time?
	drivers	sit for hours?

Note: Number of sentences that you will get will be 100.

1. *Add* **'not'** *after the subject to change them into* **Interrogative Negative**.

2. *Work with the following table to construct sentences into* **Negative**; *and to change the above sentences into* **Negative sentences**.

8. Present Indefinite (Negative)

I		work hard.
We		lead a tough life.
They	do not	show great skill.
Workers	don't	perform well.
Officers		help the society.
Players		live for others.
Writers		sense the danger in time.
Students		take safety measures.
Farmers		come in time.
Drivers		sit for hours.

Note: The maximum number of sentences that can be formed will be 200.

9. Simple Past or Past Indefinite

I	carried the load for a mile.
We	threw the baskets in the ditch.
He	placed the articles on the tables.
She	swept the vehicle.
They	polished the seats.
The cyclists	loaded the packets.

The drivers The traders The farmers The venders	crossed the city. slowed the vehicle. sold the bags. shifted the position. Opened the door. allowed only one person to sit. bought a healthy sheep. collected flowers from the backyard.

Note: You can form as many as 140 sentences, but the **Noun/Pronoun** *in the* **first person** *will keep changing—some in* **Singular Number** *and the others in* **Plural Number**.

10. Form as many sentences as you can and identify and underline the Tense of Verb in each case.

He She Krishna Sheela A hawker A vendor	gave sold sent	her him me	some honey. some money. a few eggs. one dozen mangoes. a nice puppy. a toy rabbit.

Note: You can form as many sentences as you can, but the **Noun/Pronoun** *in the first person will be in* **Singular Number**.

11. Past Imperfect or Past Continuous Tense

He	Was	singing hymns.
She		writing letters.
A worker		calling someone.
The manager		going for a walk.
A devotee		coming towards the temple.
		playing with children.
		sitting in the field.
		teaching some people.
		cleaning the table.
		arranging papers.

Note: Form as many sentences as you can but the **Noun/Pronoun** *in the first person will be in* **Singular Number** *and the maximum number of sentences that can be formed will be 50.*

12. Past Imperfect or Past Continuous Tense

He	Was	singing hymns.
She		writing letters.
A worker		calling someone.
The manager		going for a walk.
A devotee		coming towards the temple.
		playing with children.
		sitting in the field.
		teaching some people.
		cleaning the table.
		arranging papers.

Note: Use **was** *for the* **Noun/Pronoun** *in* **Singular Number** *and* **were** *for* **Plural Numbers** – *such as We, Children and They.*

13. Past Imperfect or Past Continuous Tense – Form as many sentences as you can but the nouns in the first person will be plural in number.

We	were	singing hymns.
The clerks		writing letters.
The priests		calling someone.
The reporters		going for a walk.
The women		coming towards the temple.
The children.		playing with children.
		sitting in the field.
		teaching some people.
		cleaning the table.
		arranging papers.

Note: You can make a maximum of 60 sentences. Since the **Noun/Pronoun** *in the* **first person** *are in* **Plural number**, *the verb used will be 'were'.*

14. Form as many sentences as you can and identify by underlining the Tense in each case.

She	had	finished the work.
He		accomplished all.
The golfer		accepted the guilt.
The player		fined the helpers.
The singer		punished others.
The hawker		claimed the share.

I		grown up strong.
We		visited the shrine.
Boys		completed the task.
Girls		created some space.
His pupils		controlled the crowd.
My sons		counted the flowers.
The salesmen		shown the way.
The workers		

Note: The number of sentences that you can form will be equal to 208.

15. Past Perfect Continuous Tense

I	had been	crying for the payment.
We		trying to get it done.
She		staying here for long.
They		dancing on the road.
He		begging for mercy.
The beggar		throwing stones recklessly.
The pensioner		getting closer.
The helper		seeking help.
The helpless		tearing papers.
A commoner		

Note: You can form a maximum of about 90 sentences from the above table.

16. Future Indefinite Tense

I shall	run	for an hour
We shall	play	for a prize.
They shall	go	for health.
He will	sing	for growth.
She will	stay	for a position
The teacher will	sleep	for a medal.
The tutor will	drink	in the field.
The passenger will	drive	in dress.
The player will	call	in the school.
The girls will	cry	
The clerks will		

Note: You can form as many sentences as you can, but the maximum number of sentences that you can get will be 990.

17. Future Imperfect or Future Continuous Tense

I shall		encouraging others.
We shall	be	discouraging others.
They shall		blaming others.
He will		praising others.
She will		talking in vain.
The teacher will		delivering a lecturer.
The tutor will		carrying the bag.
The passenger will		typing a letter.
The player will		starting the computer.
The girls will		watching the match.
The clerks will		buying a ticket.

Note: You can form as many sentences as you can, but the maximum number of sentences that you can get will be 121.

18. Future Perfect Tense

I	will have/shall	finished the work.
We		accomplished all.
Boys		accepted the guilt.
Girls		fined the helpers.
His pupils		punished others.
My sons		claimed the share.
The salesmen		grown up strong.
The representatives		visited the shrine.
The workers		completed the task.
She		created some space.
He		controlled the crowd.
The golfer		counted the flowers.
The player		shown the way.
The singer		
The hawker		
The shopkeeper		

Note: You can form as many sentences as you can but the maximum number of sentences that you can get will be 208.

19. Future Perfect Continuous

I shall	have been	crying for the payment.
We shall		trying to get it done.
She will		staying here for long.
They will		dancing on the road.
He will		begging for mercy.
The beggar will		throwing stones recklessly.
The pensioner will		getting closer.
The helper will		seeking help.
The helpless will		tearing papers.
A commoner will		

Note: *You can form as many sentences as you can with the* **Future Perfect Continuous Tense,** *i.e.,* **'shall or will have been'**, *but the maximum number of sentences that you can get will be 90.*

Chapter-16

Voice

Exercises

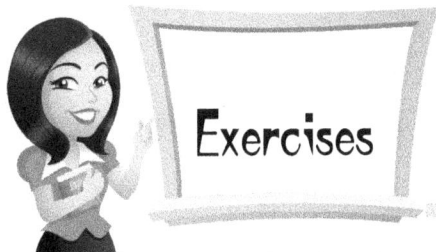

1. **Rewrite the following sentences according to the instructions given after each:**
   - ❏ The police caught the thief. (End: …. By the police)
   - ❏ Too much is being taken for granted. (Begin: They are….)
   - ❏ Who has broken the mirror? (Begin: By whom….)
   - ❏ They must do it at once. (End:… done at once.)
   - ❏ Someone has picked his pocket. (Begin: His pocket….)
   - ❏ Passengers are forbidden to cross the line. (End:…. Forbids passengers to cross the line)
   - ❏ Post this letter. (Begin: Let….)
   - ❏ They feel that these situations need never arise. (End:…. felt that these situations need never arise).
   - ❏ Will they help you? (End…. By them?)

2. **Without adding 'by'; change the following sentences into Passive Voice:**
   - ❏ Somebody built this orphanage last year.
   - ❏ People speak Hindi all over the world.
   - ❏ No one has ever achieved greatness without sincere efforts.
   - ❏ We called her stupid.
   - ❏ Someone has stolen his water heater.
   - ❏ People speak Assamese in Assam.
   - ❏ They don't like newcomers in this village.
   - ❏ They are serving cold drinks in the party.
   - ❏ They drank a whole jug of juice.
   - ❏ People always admire the brave.

3. **Change the voice of the following sentences:**
    - ❑ Open the window.
    - ❑ Her attitude shocked me a lot.
    - ❑ The farmers are ploughing their fields.
    - ❑ He landed the helicopter safely.
    - ❑ My mother was feeding the birds.
    - ❑ We are expecting rain.
    - ❑ You should follow the advice of saints.
    - ❑ Don't throw stones at the frogs.
    - ❑ Take care of your health.

4. **Change the following sentences into the Active Voice. Frame at least two sentences following the pattern of each Sentence given below.**
    - ❑ Hindi is spoken in India.
    - ❑ The letter was given to me.
    - ❑ You are requested not to cry.
    - ❑ The poor should be fed.
    - ❑ The children must be loved.
    - ❑ The goods are carried by trucks.
    - ❑ Nothing is to be gained.
    - ❑ Kites were being flown.
    - ❑ He was refused admission.
    - ❑ They are being shown how to do it.
    - ❑ This matter must be looked into.
    - ❑ It is believed that the earth is round.
    - ❑ I hope to be rewarded.
    - ❑ She was paid her wages.
    - ❑ I was helped.

❀❀❀

Chapter-17

What are Phrases and Clauses?

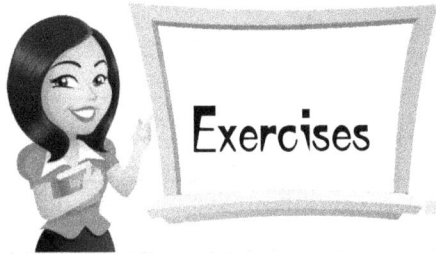

Exercises

A

1. **In each of the following sentences, replace the ADVERB in italics by an Adverb Phrase of the same meaning.**

   a. The pigeon flies *swiftly*.
      The pigeon flies _____.
   b. Did Anne behave well?
      Did Anne behave _____?
   c. Go away.
      Go _____.
   d. The dying man replied feebly.
      The dying man replied _____.
   e. Gently fell the rain.
      _____ fell the rain.
   f. We will pitch our tents just here.
      We will pitch our tents just _____.
   g. He expects to get promotion soon.
      He expects to get promotion _____.

B

1. **Some Exercises of Forming Sentences with Clauses**

	what I am going to tell you.
	all that I have to say.
Plan carefully	the things that must be known.
Listen to	the future plan.
Listen carefully	the actions of future.

Listen and follow	the blue print of the work chart.
Remember	what you have to do.
	what is needed now.
	what is important.
	what was discussed in the meeting.

Note: *The number of sentences that you form will be 24. Also identify the type of clause in each case.*

2. Form sentences and identify the type of clause in each case.

				they have done.
I	can't			they have told.
You	can	justify	what	they have achieved.
He	must	understand	that which	they have overlooked.
	must not	remind	the thing that	they have forgotten.
	should			they have borrowed.
	should not			they are overlooking.
				is important.

Note: *The number of sentences that you can get will be 756. Also identify the type of clause in each case.*

	what I am going to tell you.
	all that I have to say.
Plan carefully	the things that must be known.
Listen to	the future plan.
Listen carefully	the actions of future.
Listen and follow	the blue print of the work chart.
Remember	what you have to do.
	what is needed now.
	what is important.
	what was discussed in the meeting.

3.

He will do that	if you want.
I shall speak to him	if you ask.
You will be informed	if it is requested.
He will accept the post	if a letter is given.

They would help you	if it is offered.
He would do it	if it is proved right.
I shall oppose him	if the deadlock continues.

Note: The maximum number of sentences that you can form will be 49.

Chapter-18

The Sentence and Kinds of Sentences

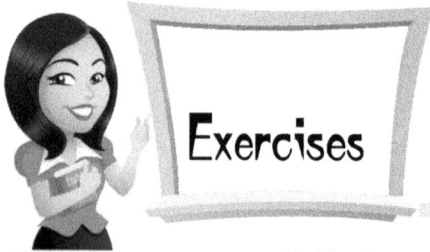

Exercises

A

1. **In the following sentences, separate the subject and the predicate.**
   - ❑ The crackling of geese saved Rome.
   - ❑ The boy stood on the burning deck.
   - ❑ Tubal Cain was a man of might.
   - ❑ Stone walls do not a prison make.
   - ❑ The singing of the birds delights us.
   - ❑ Miss kitty was rude at the table one day.
   - ❑ He has a good memory.
   - ❑ Bad habits grow unconsciously.
   - ❑ The earth revolves round the sun.
   - ❑ Nature is the best physician.

2. **Separate the subject from the predicate in the following sentences.**
   - ❑ Edison invented the phonograph.
   - ❑ The sea hath many thousand sands.
   - ❑ We cannot pump the ocean dry.
   - ❑ Borrowed garments never fit well.
   - ❑ The early bird catches the worm
   - ❑ All matter is indestructible
   - ❑ Ascham taught Latin to queen Elizabeth.
   - ❑ We should profit by experience.
   - ❑ All roads lead to Rome.

❑   A guilty conscience needs no excuse.

B

Affirmative and Negative Sentences

1. Forming of Affirmative Sentences

Match the Sentences and frame at least two Sentences of your own following the patterns.

				they have done.
I	can't			they have told.
You	can	justify	what	they have achieved.
He	must	understand	that which	they have overlooked.
	must not	remind	the thing that	they have forgotten.
	should			they have borrowed.
	should not			they are overlooking.
				is important.

Number of Sentences that you will get = 7 + 14 = 21

2. Forming of Negative Sentences

Match the sentences and frame at least two sentences of your own following the patterns.

Are you going to work?	Yes, I am.
Can you drive a car?	Yes, I can.
Does Rita sleep well?	Yes, she does.
Did he say anything?	Yes, he did.
Is it a good film?	Yes, it is.
Sheela has already come.	So, she has.
He looks unwell.	Yes, he does.

Note: *The maximum number of sentences that you will get = 7 + 14=21*

Match the sentences. Choose from the second part to complete the sentences of the first part.

Leave the room	a limping elephant.
He failed	to be very clever.
An honest man	when she was clearing the shelf.
She always wanted	and won the match.
Luckily we	when he fared well in the interview.
We saw	to be drowned in a flooded river.
Sadly he was	and they left for the show.
She seems	to become a nurse.

She fell	at 5 a.m.
He was reported	for security reasons.
We played well	put behind the bar.
We locked the gate	escaped the accident.
The rain stopped	because he acted upon your advice.
He was appointed	is always daring.

Note: The maximum number of sentences that you can get = 14

3. Match the sentences. Choose from the second part to complete the sentences of the first part.

The Mount Everest is the highest	
January is the coldest	artist.
The Ganges is a sacred	river.
Mr. Roy is a great	game.
Ludo is the funniest	peak.
Polo is a different	month.
Nainital is a very high	
December is a very cold	
May si the hottest	
Vindhya is a famous	

Note: The maximum number of sentences that you will get = 10.

4. Choose the correct Interrogative Pronoun to complete an Interrogative Sentence. Each Interrogative Pronoun will not be suitable to each given part.

	the manager of the bank?
	the eldest sister?
Who is	I ask for help?
What is	the name of the movie?
Whom should	the longest river in Asia?
Which is	the person you are talking about?
	your preference?
	we meet first?

Note: The maximum number of sentences that you will get = 8

❀❀❀

Chapter-19

Synthesis of Sentences

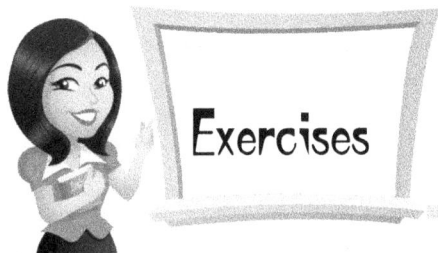

Exercises

A

1. Join the following pairs of sentences using a conjunction to form a compound sentence.

1. You must follow my instructions. You must resign.
2. John couldn't have done this. Sam couldn't have done this.
3. The burglars looted the shop. They set fire to it.
4. He is hurt. He wants to play.
5. He was very weak. He could barely stand.
6. Give me the keys of the safe. You will be shot.
7. He would not eat. He would not allow us to eat.
8. The situation is not very difficult. People think that it is very difficult.
9. The officer was very inefficient. He had to be sacked.
10. The task is very difficult. You can't do it alone.

B

1. Match the sentences and frame at least two sentences of your own following the patterns of each synthesised sentence.

After burning the midnight oil	he topped in the class.
On hearing my voice	the child ran to me.
She has four children	to support.
I have much work	to do.
This is my student	Sunny.
Nehru, a famous writer	wrote the 'Discovery of India.'
Having finished this work	the workers left for home.
Being a true patriot	he will not betray his country.

In spite of being weak	he studies hard.
Frustrated with loss in business	he went mad.
While walking on the road	I saw a big dog.
Having finished his studies	he started his own agency.
Undoubtedly,	he is a great sportsman.
They had not arrived	till now.
You are taking up old issues	unnecessarily.

Note: The number of sentences that you will get= 15 + 30=45.

2. Form Compound Sentences

Match the sentences and frame at least two sentences of your own following the patterns of each synthesised sentence.

We went to the University	and studied there.
She is a coward	and a fool.
Kiran is both	intelligent and beautiful.
Neither a borrower	nor a lender be.
Either Rajan or Ravi	will have to face the situation.
Word hard	else you will fail.
Either pay the price	or return the pen.
I know Mohan	but not Ravi.
Though, I rebuked him	yet he kept mum.
Although, he lost his position	nevertheless, he kept his cool.
I don't believe in what you say	however, I shall not oppose you.
She stood first in the class	therefore, she was given a prize.
I can't depend on him	for he is a fool.
He is definitely	talented and diligent.

Note: The maximum number of sentences you will get = 14 + 28= 32.

3   Form Complex Sentences

Match the sentences and frame at least two sentences of your own following the patterns of each synthesised sentence.

Everyone knows it	that he is an honest boy.
The fact that Bose was a great scientist	can not be challenged.
Ask him	why he is late.
I can not understand	what you say.
He is the boy	who stood first in his class.
This is the book	which he gave me.
They want a mechanic	who repairs computers.

| This is the girl | whom her mother is calling. |

Note: The maximum number of sentences formed will be 8 + 16=24.

Chapter-20

Transformation of Sentences

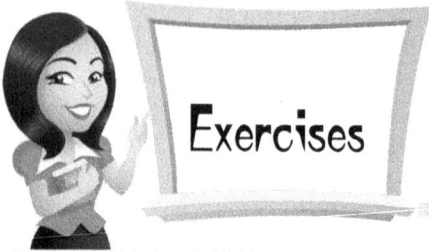

Exercises

1. **Interchange the principal and the subordinate clauses in the following sentences:**
   - ❏ Look before you leap.
   - ❏ As soon as the storm began, the boat capsized.
   - ❏ Unless you work hard, you will not come up in life.
   - ❏ He never makes a promise which he cannot keep.
   - ❏ He ran away as soon as he saw me.
   - ❏ I cannot speak loudly because I have a sore throat.
   - ❏ I was so foolish that I did not act upon my teacher's advice.
   - ❏ She does not like him because he is proud.
   - ❏ No sooner did the bell ring than the boys ran into their classes.
   - ❏ The money was not returned until the thief was beaten.

❖❖❖

Chapter-21

Direct and Indirect Speech

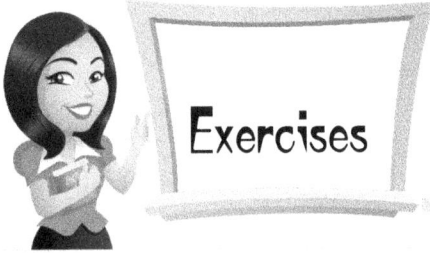

Exercises

A

1. **Rewrite the following in Direct Speech:**
   - ❑ The boy asked me how old I was.
   - ❑ The stranger asked Ashish where he lived.
   - ❑ Ramu asked Nitin whether he had made a mistake.
   - ❑ They asked me what I wanted.
   - ❑ The young mouse asked who would bell the cat.
   - ❑ I asked Nihal if he would lend me a pen.
   - ❑ The policeman inquired of the girl where she was going.
   - ❑ She enquired of us whether we were playing football.

B

1. **Form ten sentences of Direct Speech. Subject + Verb+ Direct Object + Preposition + Prepositional Object**

Thank	You	for	your kind help.
Ask	him	for	a few more.
Compare	this	with	that flag.
They punished	him	for	being very late.
Congratulate	him	on	his grand success.
Do not throw	the stone	at	the poor donkey.
What prevented	you	from	joining the post?

Add	this	to	what you have.
I explained	my difficulty	to	the manager.
Protect	us	from	the terrorists.

Note: The maximum number of sentences that you will get is 10.

2. Form Indirect Sentences. Subject + Verb + Indirect Object + Direct Object

Subject + Verb	Indirect Object	Direct Object
Have they paid	You	the subscription?
Will you lend	me	your book?
Did our teacher give	us	home work?
Did I read	him	the newspaper?
Please throw	me	a pen.
His grand father told	him	a nice story.
He handed	me	the cheque.
The pupils wished	the teachers	'Happy New Year.'
He denies	her	nothing essential.

Note: The maximum number of sentences that you will get is 9.

✤✤✤

Chapter-22

Punctuation

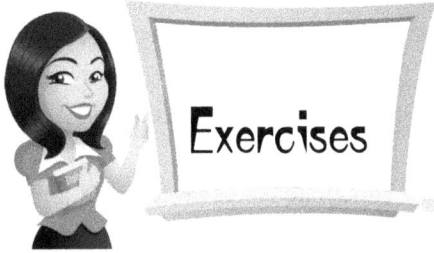

Exercises

This exercise will test your understanding of all kinds of different punctuation marks, particularly, *commas, colons, semi-colons and apostrophes.*

Select the correctly punctuated sentence by putting a tick mark _____ on the right one.

1. a) Spain is a beautiful country; the beache's are warm, sandy and spotlessly clean.
   b) Spain is a beautiful country: the beaches are warm, sandy and spotlessly clean.
   c) Spain is a beautiful country, the beaches are warm, sandy and spotlessly clean.
   d) Spain is a beautiful country; the beaches are warm, sandy and spotlessly clean.

2. a) The children's books were all left in the following places: Mrs Smith's room, Mr. Powell's office and the caretaker's cupboard.
   b) The children's books were all left in the following places; Mrs Smith's room, Mr Powell's office and the caretaker's cupboard.
   c) The childrens books were all left in the following places: Mrs Smiths room, Mr Powells office and the caretakers cupboard.
   d) The children's books were all left in the following places, Mrs Smith's room, Mr Powell's office and the caretaker's cupboard.

3. a) She always enjoyed sweets, chocolate, marshmallows and toffee apples.
   b) She always enjoyed: sweets, chocolate, marshmallows and toffee apples.
   c) She always enjoyed sweets chocolate marshmallows and toffee apples.
   d) She always enjoyed sweet's, chocolate, marshmallow's and toffee apple's.

4. a) Sarah's uncle's car was found without its wheels in that old derelict warehouse.
   b) Sarah's uncle's car was found without its wheels in that old, derelict warehouse.
   c) Sarahs uncles car was found without its wheels in that old, derelict warehouse.
   d) Sarah's uncle's car was found without it's wheels in that old, derelict warehouse.

5. a) I can't see Tim's car, there must have been an accident.
   b) I cant see Tim's car; there must have been an accident.
   c) I can't see Tim's car there must have been an accident.
   d) I can't see Tim's car; there must have been an accident.

6. a) Paul's neighbours were terrible; so his brother's friends went round to have a word.
   b) Paul's neighbours were terrible: so his brother's friends went round to have a word.
   c) Paul's neighbours were terrible, so his brother's friends went round to have a word.
   d) Paul's neighbours were terrible so his brother's friends went round to have a word.

7. a) Tims gran, a formidable woman, always bought him chocolate, cakes, sweets and a nice fresh apple.
   b) Tim's gran a formidable woman always bought him chocolate, cakes, sweets and a nice fresh apple.
   c) Tim's gran, a formidable woman, always bought him chocolate cakes sweets and a nice fresh apple.
   d) Tim's gran, a formidable woman, always bought him chocolate, cakes, sweets and a nice fresh apple.

8. a) After stealing Tims car, the thief lost his way and ended up the chief constable's garage.
   b) After stealing Tim's car the thief lost his way and ended up the chief constable's garage.
   c) After stealing Tim's car, the thief lost his way and ended up the chief constable's garage.
   d) After stealing Tim's car, the thief lost his' way and ended up the chief constable's garage.

9. a) We decided to visit: Spain, Greece, Portugal and Italy's mountains.
   b) We decided to visit Spain, Greece, Portugal and Italys mountains.
   c) We decided to visit Spain, Greece, Portugal and Italy's mountains.
   d) We decided to visit Spain Greece Portugal and Italy's mountains.

10. a) That tall man, Paul's grandad, is this month's winner.
    b) That tall man Paul's grandad is this month's winner.
    c) That tall man, Paul's grandad, is this months winner.
    d) That tall man, Pauls grandad, is this month's winner.

❧❧❧

Chapter-23

Idioms

Exercises

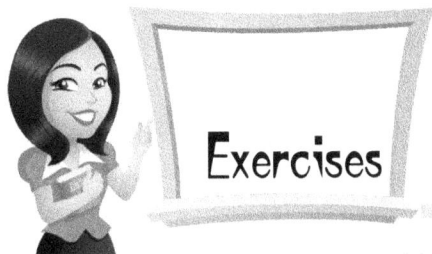

1. Choose the correct meaning of the Idiom from the Four Options given in each case.

1. **To end in smoke**
   - ❏ Smoking too many cigarettes
   - ❏ Face failure
   - ❏ House burnt down
   - ❏ Religious ceremony

2. **To get into hot waters**
   - ❏ Bathe in the winter months
   - ❏ To get rich
   - ❏ To get healthy
   - ❏ To get into trouble

3. **To make ends meet**
   - ❏ A short story
   - ❏ To skip classes
   - ❏ To earn enough to live
   - ❏ To be an expert

4. **Bolt from the blue**
   - ❏ Sudden shock
   - ❏ To lose a tight game
   - ❏ To get punched
   - ❏ To ask for help

5. **To burn the candle at both ends**
   - ❏ To argue endlessly
   - ❏ To work long hours
   - ❏ Long power cut
   - ❏ To have a good time

6. **To bury the hatchet**
   - ❏ To end enmity
   - ❏ To hide stolen treasure
   - ❏ To kill someone
   - ❏ To overexert

7. **To spill the beans**
   - ❏ To eat clumsily
   - ❏ To get exhausted
   - ❏ To reveal a secret
   - ❏ To fight

8. **To lead someone up the garden path**
   - ❏ To give directions
   - ❏ To mislead someone
   - ❏ To show a beautiful place
   - ❏ To exaggerate

9. **To weather a storm**
   - ❏ To criticise someone
   - ❏ To be an introvert
   - ❏ To survive a crisis
   - ❏ To guess correctly

10. **To bite one's lip**
    - ❏ To be unsure
    - ❏ To not react despite being angry
    - ❏ To feel sorry at someone's plight
    - ❏ To laugh at someone's misfortune

2. Choose the correct meaning of the Idiom in each case from the given options.

1. **What does the idiom 'to foam at one's mouth' mean?**

   a) to get very angry

   b) To brush vigorously so that foam forms in your mouth.

   c) To salivate on seeing food

2. **To 'feel like a fish out of water' is to feel**

   a) unhappy

   b) uncomfortable

   c) angry

   d) dejected

3. **When something is done at the eleventh hour, it is done**

   a) too early

   b) too late

   c) immediately

   d) at the last minute

4. **What do you mean when you say you have burnt your fingers?**

   a) that you have suffered financial losses

   b) that you have got hurt physically

   c) that you have to find work

   d) that you have just had a miraculous escape

5. **What do you mean by the idiom 'add fuel to fire'?**

   a) to say or do something that would make a bad situation even worse

   b) to investigate something

c) to initiate something

d) none of these

6. **What does the idiom 'off the top of your head' mean?**

   a) to say something without thinking much

   b) to do something that would put you in trouble

   c) to act recklessly

   d) none of these

Answers

A-1 (1) Face failure (2) To get into trouble (3) To earn enough to live (4) Sudden shock, (5) To work long hours (6) To end enmity (7) To reveal a secret (8) To mislead someone (9) To survive a crisis (10) To not react despite being angry.

A-2 (1) To get very angry (2) To feel uncomfortable (3) It is done too late (4) That you have suffered financial losses (5) to say or do something that would make a bad situation even worse (6) To say something without thinking much

Chapter-24

Phrases, Proverbs and Expressions

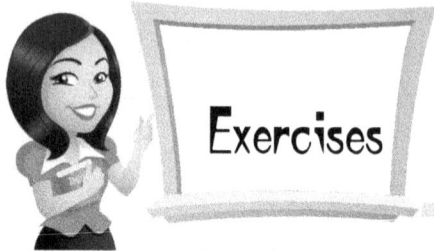

Exercises

Identify and Underline the Phrases/Proverbs in the following sentences.

1.

- ❑ Today he is in high spirits.
- ❑ Prohibition is gall and wormwood to distillers.
- ❑ The screen is in character with the rest of the furniture.
- ❑ I am afraid I am in his bad books.
- ❑ The thief took to his heels on seeing a policeman

2.

- ❑ He keeps in touch with the latest developments in wireless.
- ❑ The scheme appears worthless at the first blush.
- ❑ I smell a rat.
- ❑ He changed colour when I questioned him about his antecedents.
- ❑ I took him to task for his carelessness.

3.

- ❑ Naturally he fights shy of his young nephew, who is a gambler.
- ❑ The old man is hard of hearing.
- ❑ I trusted him and he played me false.
- ❑ I am out of pocket by the transaction.
- ❑ He is working against time.

4.

- [ ] I am afraid he is burning the candles at both ends.
- [ ] Late in life he tried his hand at farming.
- [ ] Throughout his speech the boys were all ears.
- [ ] While he was speaking his father cut him short.
- [ ] Stick to your colours, my boys!

5.

- [ ] A dispute in a south Wales colliery came to a head.
- [ ] He is rather blunt, but his heart is in the right place.
- [ ] I did not notice in him anything out of the way.
- [ ] In the contest he came off second-best.
- [ ] The usurper cannot maintain his position without the sinews of war.
- [ ]

Chapter-25

Miscellaneous Exercises

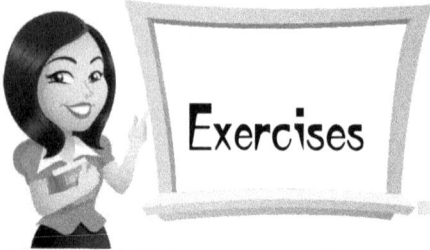

Exercises

Exercise 1

Write the sentences and frame at least two sentences of your own following the pattern of each Sentence.

		the large red ball.
He	took out	the long yellow.
She	put down	the small green book.
Sweta	picked up	a white cricket ball.
Seema	rubbed with	a sharp knife.
Shashi	threw away	a steel pan.

Number of sentences = 150 + 300

Exercise 2

Write the sentences and frame at least two sentences of your own following the pattern of each sentence.

They worked	all the day.
They played	throughout the morning.
They worshipped God	during the evening.
They sang hymns	from two o'clock.
They performed sacrifices	from six o'clock till noon.
He meditated	for two hours.
He practised yoga	from ten thirty sharp.
She looked after the guests	for many days.
They learnt lessons	until two o'clock.

The manager searched the file	till the evening.
The lady remained engaged	From eleven AM to 3 PM.

Number of sentences = 121 + 242

Exercise 3

Write the sentences and frame at least two sentences of your own following the pattern of each sentence.

The sun always rises	
The sun never sets	in the east.
The sun shines	during the day.
The students go to school	during the morning hours.
Everything shines	with a hope.
A lot of knowledge comes first	faithfully.
All the light is scattered first	

Number of sentences = 35 + 70

Exercise 4

Write the Sentences and frame at least two Sentences of your own following the pattern of each Sentence.

I write Aum, the symbol of Brahma	
We eat something	every Thursday.
We visit the temple	every morning.
We have lessons	once everyday.
They clean the shop	thrice daily.
He works at a hall and goes there	without fail.
We play the tabala	regularly.
We take lessons in music	

Number of sentences = 48 + 96

Exercise 5

Write the sentences and frame at least two sentences of your own following the pattern of each sentence.

			been to Varanasi.
He has	once		been up in an airplane.
There are people that have	often		seen women fighting.
All philanthropic persons have	twice		found courageous faring well.
These worshippers have	never		helped the poor and needy.

		been selected in the preliminary.
		encountered true devotees.

Number of sentences = 112 +224

Exercise 6

Write the sentences and frame at least two sentences of your own following the pattern of each sentence.

There are still some green trees	
There must be fruit trees	in all regions.
We must plant and protect trees	along the sides of the roads.
They have deputed volunteers	in each garden and field.
They are arranging free feasts	At vacant places
They drew some demarcating lines	
There are heaps of garbage	

Number of sentences = 28 + 56

Exercise 7

Write the sentences and frame at least two sentences of your own following the pattern of each sentence.

Shekhar spends a lot	on books.
Mr Sinha spends a lot of time	on study.
She spends very little money	on tuition.
Mr. Thakur spends nothing	on healthy growth.
I have been regularly spending something	on junk food.
Everyone must spend	on fresh vegetables.

Number of sentences = 36 + 72

Exercise 8

Write (a) answers to the questions; and (b) change them into affirmative sentences.

Is the man with white cap sitting or standing?
What is the man with an iron ladder doing?
Why is the sound of the machine is not coming?
Why is the printer taking many pages at a time?
What colour is the shirt that I gave you yesterday?
Where did you keep the attendance register?
Where can I get a few boxes of white chalk?

English Grammar Workbook

Why did she give you a hard pencil?
Where did you buy that green book with yellow pages?
How can the long holidays be happily spent?

Number of sentences = 10 + 20

Exercise 9

Write the sentences and frame at least two sentences of your own following the pattern of each sentence.

I have not finished the drawing yet.
I'm still drawing the body.
I have already drawn the eyes.
She has placed many flowers in the vessel.
Some of the flowers are yellow and some are white.
Now, there are enough flowers in the pot.
Yet, some more flowers can be added to it.
The pot is too full to hold any more.
She poured water into the pot but not much.
A little work and the pot has increased the beauty many times.

Number of sentences 10 + 20

Exercise 10

Write the sentences and frame at least two sentences of your own following the pattern of each sentence.

She hit herself with the roller.
While cutting vegetables you yourself have injured your fingers.
I must blame myself for coming late.
One must feel the burden of responsibility on oneself.
We have tried hard to start the machine ourselves.
He himself dug his grave by allowing aliens to live with him.
They themselves assembled the complete computer set.
The plate itself slipped down from the rack.

Number of sentences 8 + 16

Exercise 11

    I.   Frame at least one sentence with each weak and strong verb.

    II.   Read, understand, learn and imbibe all the weak and strong verbs and keep them on the tip of tongue and pen. One can't learn English without having command of V1, V2 and V3.

III. Read a book on English Grammar from page one to the last and solve all the exercises given in it. The reading of the total book without leaving anything out will give you a complete picture of English language. Never think of important and unimportant chapters. Everything and all the chapters are important. If they are not important then they would not have been there.

IV. Remember to write a complete sentence every time. Don't write one part many times then the other part that many time to show to the teacher of guardian that you have completed the task. It is not solving task, it is learning.

V. Complete sentences will give 'completeness' to your knowledge and ability.

VI. Writing many pages a day will bear fruits in their own way, according to their capacity but they are bound to teach you. Remember: Reading makes a wise man; speaking makes a ready man but writing makes a perfect man.

VII. Frame sentences of your own: as many as you can within the available time limit. It will give command over spelling and punctuation. This practice from an early age will bear immense sweet fruits later on during maturity when all the sentence pattern are a part and parcel of consciousness.

VIII. Always keep a handy Dictionary at hand. Collect and obtain mastery over the words. Remember: there are neither easy words nor difficult words; words are either known or unknown; and they help.

IX. Remember your God; have patience, courage and confidence; and go ahead. You are the winner.

Prepositions, Clauses and Others

1. Prepositions

	apple tree				
	ox				
An	owl	is	in	the	field.
	onion carton	was	around		garden.
	orange-box				hut.
	elephant				house.
	old woman				
	oil-can				

Number of sentences = 128

2. Prepositions

An officer	came	to me.
An official messenger	came fast	to her house.
An agent	was coming	from the southern end.
An old car	was not coming	with some papers.

An air courier	did not come	on an urgent mission.
An applicant	will come	for consultation.
	will not come	Without an appointment.

Number of sentences = 294

3. Prepositions

The book		on the table.
The pen		in the bag.
The pencil	is	in the box.
The copy	was	in the drawer.
The diary	will be	at the top of the almirah.
The register	is not	behind the rack.
The key	was not	by the books.
The file	will not be	under the table
The pictures		under the chair.
The watch		beside the mirror.

Number of sentences = 600

4. Prepositions

The book			on the table.
The pen			in the bag.
The pencil	is	kept	in the box.
The copy	was	lying	in the drawer.
The diary	will be		at the top of the almirah.
The register	is not		behind the rack.
The key	was not		by the books.
The file	will not be		under the table
The pictures			under the chair.
The watch			beside the mirror.

Number of sentences = 1200

5. Prepositions

They		in	India.
The technicians	fought	for	the University.
The employees	called a strike	out of	the factory.

The people	created a scene	against	

Number of sentences = 194

6. Prepositions

The book		above my head.
The pen		above my shoulder.
The pencil	has been	by the wall.
The copy	had been	by the rack.
The diary	has been lying	without cover.
The register	had been lying	out of sight.
The key	has not been lying	out of my reach.
The file	had not been lying	before me.
The pictures		behind the librarian.
The watch		on the shelf.

Number of sentences = 600

7. Prepositions

He		waiting for a bus.
She		planning to go on a picnic.
Rajesh	is	working for many years.
Zafar	was	earning a lot of money.
My mother	has been	walking without a stick.
Her sister	had been	roaming on foot.
Your uncle	will be	running with an aim.
The manager		speaking in a meeting.

Number of sentences = 284

8. Prepositions

		working with a motive.
		writing for a magazine.
We	are	looking for a job.
They	were	running around.
You	have been	moving from pillar to post.
	had been	switching off the lights.
	will be	pulling it up.
	will not be	throwing that down.
		relaxing on the sofa.

		lying by the wall.
		waiting at the ticket window.
		arriving in time.
		present in the meeting.

Number of sentences = 234

9. Prepositions

I have		for two months.
You have	lived here	for several years.
He has	worked there	for a long time.
She has	studied Grammar	for three years.
My friend has	been a lecturer	since 2005.
They have	practised as a doctor	since June last.
		since last Diwali.

Number of sentences = 210

10. Prepositions

All the		are walking	to the pond.
Both the	boys	walked	to the swimming pool.
Some of the	girls	will walk	to the market.
The other	persons	are going	to the book fair.
Some	students	went	away from the exhibition.
Five		will go	across the field.

Number of sentences = 576

11. Prepositions

He earns his living by	working in the factory.
He can establish peace by	strengthening union.
Mohan is fond of	learning languages.
Priya is clever at	teaching in a school.
Gita is interested in	singing religious songs.
Deepa has strong plea for	performing dances.
He became rich after	getting a good job.
He got money without	maintaining communal harmony.
You can do nothing without	

Number of sentences = 72

12. Prepositions

Sita,		these pens	
Ramesh,		this box	in your desk.
Rajesh,	please, put	that book	on my table.
Lipika,		these shirts	near the window.
Tanu,		the album	behind the door.
		the painting	

Number of sentences = 120

13. Prepositions

The nail			the table.
The hammer		in front of	the wardrobe.
The axe	is	behind	the show case.
The knife	was	in the middle of	the rack.
The nail-file		at the top of	the rack.
The rod		at the bottom of	the board.
The duster			the pot.
The medicine			the box.

Number of sentences = 768

14. Prepositions

There is a nice picture	in the hall.
There is a big desk	by the wall.
There is a small table	on the floor.
There are three black boxes	at the door.
There are four new chairs	in the truck.
There are five long benches	between the table.

15.

I	always	look at the pictures.
You	seldom	look through the window.
They	often	look down upon the misers.
The boys	usually	go home early.
		complete works in time.
		get up early.
		play football.

		read stories.
		prepare the lessons.

16.

'An apple for an apple'	
'An eye for an eye'	is the dictum.
'All is well that ends well'	is true for all time.
'He that leaps will fall'	is a famous proverb.
'Better late than never'	is the saying of wise men.
'Charity begins at home'	

Number of sentences = 24

17. Clauses

	what I am going to tell you.
	all that I have to say.
Plan carefully	the things that must be known.
Listen to	the future plan.
Listen carefully	the actions of future.
Listen and follow	the blue print of the work chart.
Remember	what you have to do.
	what is needed now.
	what is important.
	what was discussed in the meeting.

Number of sentences = 24

18. Clauses

				they have done.
I	can't			they have told.
You	can	justify	what	they have achieved.
He	must	understand	that which	they have overlooked.
	must not	remind	the thing that	they have forgotten.
	should			they have borrowed.
	should not			they are overlooking.
				is important.

Number of sentences = 756

19. Clauses

He will do that	if you want.
I shall speak to him	if you ask.
You will be informed	if it is requested.
He will accept the post	if a letter is given.
They would help you	if it is offered.
He would do it	if it is proved right.
I shall oppose him	if the deadlock continues.

Number of sentences = 49

20.

		bite.
I	continued to	come.
You	began to	speak.
They	used to	strike hard.
He		look down upon.
She		spend a lot.
People		read everything.
Boys		play only football.
		make a car.
		sing well.
		swim for a long time.
		shed tears.
		tell lies.
		throw away the money.

Number of sentences = 252

21.

I		breaking wood.
We	went on	going ahead.
You	kept on	singing songs.
He	started	reciting rhymes.
She		drinking cold water.
They		giving instructions.
People		telling a story.
Boys		reading poems.
Girls		running fast.

Number of sentences = 243

English Grammar Workbook

22.

I	informed		the banker will call at your place.
He	intimated	that	Sita was called for an explanation.
She	told the news		the doctor was called in time.
We	gave the information		the strike was called off.
They			the culprit was brought to book.
			they brought about their own ruin.

Number of sentences = 144

23.

Praveen	Called the doctor in.
They	Threw the ball away.
We	Cut the ribbon off.
I	Sent them back.
You	Put the gown on.
He	Called the strike off.
She	Put off the lamp.
Seema	Gave away the prizes.
The President	Was hit for three consecutive sixes.
His uncle	Foolishly played with flames.
Her brother	Looked into the matter.
My sister	Will abide by the rules.
	Will take care of the expenses.
	Will not stop in the middle.
	Will freely work for the children.

Number of sentences = 180

24. Comparisons

	pen			
This	book		charming	as that.
	watch	is as	beautiful	
	horse	is not as	pretty	
	house	is not so	useful	
	car		useless	

	curtain		dirty	
	office		pleasant	
	drawer		refreshing	
	incense			
	perfume			

Number of sentences = 264

25. Comparisons

	pen			
This	book	is more	charming	as that.
	watch	is less	beautiful	
	horse		pretty	
	house		useful	
	car		useless	
	curtain		dirty	
	office		pleasant	
	drawer		refreshing	
	incense			
	perfume			

Number of sentences = 176

26. Comparisons

	pen			
This	book	is the most	charming	of all.
	watch	is the least	beautiful	
	horse		pretty	
	house		useful	
	car		useless	
	curtain		dirty	
	office		pleasant	
	drawer		refreshing	
	incense			
	perfume			

Number of sentences = 176

English Grammar Workbook

27. Comparisons

This young man This boy This rich man This merchant This river This leader This manager	is as is not as is not so	idle truthful wicked popular greedy famous dangerous	as that.

Number of sentences = 147

28. Comparisons

This young man This boy This rich man This merchant This river This leader This manager	is more is less	idle truthful wicked popular greedy famous dangerous	as that.

Number of sentences = 147

29. Comparisons

This young man This boy This rich man This merchant This river This leader This manager	is the most is the least	idle truthful wicked popular greedy famous dangerous	as that.

Number of sentences = 147

30. Comparisons

This leader			
This pleader		greater	than that.
This teacher	is	wiser	
This young man	was	cleverer	
This boy	will be	truer	
This rich man		more popular	
This merchant		more learned	
This river		more honest	
This leader		more diligent	
This manager			

Number of sentences = 240

31. Comparisons

This leader			
This pleader		the greatest	of all.
This teacher	is	the wisest	
This young man	was	the most successful	
This boy	will be	the most worthy	
This rich man		more popular	
This merchant		more learned	
This river		more honest	
This leader		more diligent	
This manager			

Number of sentences = 240

32. Narration

He says We know She fears You think He will say I say You hear	that	he is ill. he goes to school. he will go to school. Mohan has done that. Mohan will do that. the boy comes late. the boy would come late. the birds are flying. the earth moves round the sun. an empty vessel sounds much. Ram killed Ravana. labour never goes in vain. honesty is the best policy.

Number of sentences = 91

33. Narration

He said I said You said We said They informed The teacher said Meera told Seema was informed They learnt	that	he would help. he would go there the next day. he has won the race. they were guilty. I was wrong. he was tired. she was very wicked. they were ready to help. the sun rises in the east. Ram was a student. Jaya was a scholar.

Number of Sentences 99

34.

I made I forced We must not let We saw I heard We watched	him her them	do it. do the work. take rest here. behave so badly. carry the box. return the loan.

Number of sentences = 108

35.

It is not necessary There is no cause It is not too late It is difficult It is very easy It is not easy	for me to walk to the office. for you to wait. for the children to play. for you to do this. for anyone to control him. for me to let him go. for me to the interest. for them to fight like this.

Number of sentences = 48

36.

We feel like We have started Don't give up I don't mind She likes I love Gopal prefers He prefers Lata enjoys They relish	playing tennis. helping others. playing harmonium and flute. dancing. working in the garden. ding outdoor works. painting portraits. taking notes. solving spiritual problems. showing compassion.

Number of sentences = 100

37.

I They We He She Raman Sarita	kept on	working moving running looking serving showing writing	and	he she Kamal Kavita the boys the girls	continued to	drink. eat. watch. play. run. read. speak.

Number of sentences = 1658

38.

This is Please give I want They bought He donated	a piece of ten metres of	cloth. rod. bamboo. wire. glass sheet. curtain.

Number of sentences = 60

39.

Please give me I gave her He offered I bought They are purchasing	a cup of a kilo of	tea. coffee. sugar. ice-cream. fruit juice honey.

Number of sentences = 108

40.

He She Ravi Ramesh Pankaj Neeraj	is	sitting running waiting moving walking	next to	Ram Kishore Mohan Dheeraj

Number of sentences = 120

41.

I You They We	want like	to collect to buy to give to show	this picture. that pen. these bottles. those cards. ripe mangoes. magnetic chess. new Dictionaries.

Number of sentences = 256

42.

He She	likes wants	to collect to buy to give to show	this arrangement. that movie. these cartoon. fresh apples. ripe mangoes. magnet. new books

Number of sentences = 112

43.

I want to know Tell me I enquired I asked him I don't know	"What is your name?" Why are you angry?" "Where do you live?" "When will you finish the work?" "Why are you ill?" "Who will feed you?" "What have you eaten?" "When did you come here?"

Number of sentences = 40

44.

I want to know Tell me I enquired I asked him I don't know	what his name was. why he was angry. where he lives. when he would finish the work. why he was ill. who will feed him. what he had eaten. when he came there.

Number of sentences = 40

45.

He She The manager The clerk	is was	believed considered proved known	to be	innocent. honest. wise. wrong. true.

46.

He The servant The girl The tall man	was	told called forced ordered asked allowed	to open the window. to be late. to arrange the articles. to carry the boxes. to clean the room. to participate in the function. to collect the scattered books. to distribute the cards.

Number of sentences = 192

47.

He She I	was	kept found seen watched	waiting working giving orders leaving the station standing outside carrying boxes cleaning the office	by her son. for her. by the boss.

Number of sentences = 360

48.

The box The door The room The locker The drawer	was	found empty. painted green. dirty. left open. thoroughly cleaned.

Number of sentences = 25

49.

Had he been	told warned reminded satisfied	that	he was mistaken he would be late he must come here early nothing could be done the plan was useless he has a meeting	?

Number of sentences = 24

Miscellaneous Exercises

50.

He was We were You were Students were	shown told advised	how to do it. when to start. how to frame sentences. which one to select. what to take. where to go. what to leave behind.

Number of sentences = 84

51.

The man who was	running fast driving a car sitting behind me	asked me to run. called me to say something. was looking pale was not known to me. had gone mad. will come again. gave me his visiting card.

Number of sentences = 84

52. Phrases

The negotiations will be finished	in a mysterious way.
I shall see you	before long.
He will get everything	without delay.
We will get a refusal	in black and white.
The plan will be discussed	right or wrong.
The situation will improve	in no time.

Number of sentences = 36

53.

The negotiations will be finished	in a mysterious way.
I shall see you	before long.
He will get everything	without delay.
We will get a refusal	in black and white.
The plan will be discussed	right or wrong.
The situation will improve obviously	in no time.

Number of sentences = 36

54.

	the face of	the clock.
	the front of	the water heater.
This is	the back of	the reservoir.
That is	the top of	the thermos.
	the bottom of	the swimming pool.

Number of sentences = 50

55.

		the maps.
These are		the charts.
Those are	the sides of	the black board.
		The box.

Number of sentences = 8

56.

		contented.
Everybody	feels	happy.
Each one of us	seems	sad.
He	looks	satisfied.
Ravi	appears to be	dissatisfied.

Number of sentences = 80

57.

		comes here.
He	hardly	seeps well.
She	generally	visits me.
Rita	some times	comes to my place.
Mohan	often	eats happily.
The boy	never	plays outside.
The girl	usually	sings songs.

Number of sentences = 84

58.

		very interesting.
The news	is	very surprising.
The result		much admired.
The invitation	was	conveyed in time.
		published in advance.
		shocking.

Number of sentences = 36

59.

		lying on the back.
I	love	to lie on grass.
We	hate	to rise up in early morning.
They	prefer	to work during afternoon.
My brothers		sitting on hard chairs.
My friends		to sit on a cushioned sofa.
		to burst out laughing.
		to spend money.
		to waste time.

Number of sentences = 165

60.

	went there	
	did it	
We	inaugurated it	yesterday.
He They	finished the book	last June.
	completed the work	two days ago.
	raised the pillar	last month.
	made a platform	

Number of sentences = 56

61.

Each of them Everyone Neither of them Either of them One of the girls Either he or she Neither he nor she	is was	rewarded. present. tall. absent. refined. cultured. diligent. intelligent. talented.

Number of sentences = 126

62.

The prisoner The father The teacher The farmer The inspector The officer	is was	angry with his son. angry at what he had heard. pleased with his performance. interested in the story. disillusioned about the future. affected by the turn of events. accused of partiality.

Number of sentences = 84

63.

Add sign of Interrogation in the Interrogative sentences.

There's There is Is there There isn't There is not	a lot of much	ink in the bottle. Water in the river. Juice in the jug. Sugar in this bag. Money in his wallet. Sand near the bank of the river.

Number of sentences = 60

64.

		match sticks in the match boxes.
There are	a few	books on the book shelf.
Are there	many	flowers in my garden.
There are not		flowering plants in my area.
		leaves on trees during winter.
		bags in the store.

Number of sentences = 36

65.

Please assist	him	to lift the suitcase.
She will help	her	to clean the cupboard.
I want	Shekhar	to bring down the iron stair.
Raman will go with		to adjust the freeze.

Number of sentences = 48

66. Phrases

He was beaten	in front of me.
He supported you	to get imaginary favour.
He was defeated	on account of ill-health.
He was victimised	in spite of hard labour.
He surrendered	owing to bad weather.
He left the job	against his will.

Number of sentences = 36

67.

		one.
	another	pen.
Here is		book.
There is		picture on page 51.
I have seen		map on the wall.
		beggar at the mosque.
		field of onion.
		set of tools.
		place for carpenters.
		mango orchard.

English Grammar Workbook

Number of sentences = 30

68.

Did you know	what	this is	called?
Can they tell		coal	used for?
Did she explain		glucose	made up of?
Can scientists analyse			

Number of sentences = 12+12 = 24

69.

I saw	the tallest tree.
They visited	the most beautiful city.
They live near	the highest mountain.
We are very close to	the oldest person.
We can't go to	the longest field.
	the largest stadium.
	the biggest market.

Number of sentences = 35

Exercise 1 - Compound Sentences

Match the sentences and frame at least two sentences of your own following the patterns of each synthesised sentence.

After burning the midnight oil	he topped in the class.
On hearing my voice	the child ran to me.
She has four children	to support.
I have much work	to do.
This is my student	Sunny.
Nehru, a famous writer	wrote the 'Discovery of India.'
Having finished this work	the workers left for home.
Being a true patriot	he will not betray his country.
In spite of being weak	he studies hard.
Frustrated with loss in business	he went mad.
While walking on the road	I saw a big dog.
Having finished his studies	he started his own agency.
Undoubtedly,	he is a great sportsman.
They had not arrived	till now.
You are taking up old issues	unnecessarily.

Number of sentences = 15 + 2 = 17

Exercise 2-Compound Sentences

Match the sentences and frame at least two sentences of your own following the patterns of each Synthesised Sentence.

We went to the University	and studied there.
She is a coward	and a fool.
Kiran is both	intelligent and beautiful.
Neither a borrower	nor a lender be.
Either Rajan or Ravi	will have to face the situation.
Word hard	else you will fail.
Either pay the price	or return the pen.
I know Mohan	but not Ravi.
Though, I rebuked him	yet he kept mum.
Although, he lost his position	nevertheless, he kept his cool.
I don't believe in what you say	however, I shall not oppose you.
She stood first in the class	therefore, she was given a prize.
I can't depend on him	for he is a fool.
He is definitely	talented and diligent.

Number of sentences = 14 + 2 = 16

Exercise 3 - Complex Sentences

Match the sentences and frame at least two sentences of your own following the patterns of each Synthesised Sentence.

Everyone knows it	that he is an honest boy.
The fact that Bose was a great scientist	can not be challenged.
Ask him	why he is late.
I can not understand	what you say.
He is the boy	who stood first in his class.
This is the book	which he gave me.
They want a mechanic	who repairs computers.
This is the girl	whom her mother is calling.

Number of Sentences = 8 + 2 = 10

Exercise 4 - Simple Answers: Affirmative

Match the sentences and frame at least two sentences of your own following the patterns given below.

Are you going to work?	Yes, I am.
Can you drive a car?	Yes, I can.
Does Rita sleep well?	Yes, she does.
Did he say anything?	Yes, he did.
Is it a good film?	Yes, it is.
Sheela has already come.	So, she has.
He looks unwell.	Yes, he does.

Number of sentences = 7 + 7 + 2 + 2 = 18

Exercise 5 - Simple Answers: Negative

Match the sentences and frame at least two sentences of your own following the patterns given below.

Are you going to work?	No, I am not.
Can you drive a car?	No, I can't.
Does Rita sleep well?	No, she does not.
Did he say anything?	No, he didn't.
Is it a good film?	No, it is not.
Sheela has already come.	No, she has not.
He looks unwell.	No, he does not.

Number of sentences = 7 + 7 + 2 + 2 = 18

Exercise 6 - Simple Answers

Match the sentences and frame at least two sentences of your own following the patterns given below.

The apples are not good.	No, they are not.
She doesn't like fish.	No, she does not.
He can't help laughing.	No, he can't.
He is unwell.	No, he is not.
You are joking.	Oh no, I'm not.
Why did you beat him?	But I didn't.
You can't understand.	Yes, I can.
He won't come again.	But he will.
You don't know him.	Oh yes, I do.

Number of sentences = 9 + 9 + 2 + 2 = 22

Exercise 7 - Frame at least five sentences of your own following the patterns given below.

Stop talking.
Sit here.
Don't talk.
Be silent.
Please give me a glass of milk.
Open the window.
Shut the door.
May he live a hundred years!
May God save the earth.

Exercise 8 - Frame at least two sentences of your own following the patterns given below.

Hush! Don't disturb the class.
Alas! My friend has met with an accident.
Hurrah! They have won the match.
Bravo! We are going to Goa next week.
Ah! He is dead.
May he survive this crisis!
If only I were a scholar!
What a nice day!
How stupid of you to behave like this!
What a fool you are!
Oh! I'm having a terrible pain in stomach.

Exercise 9 - (Voice) Frame at least five sentences (Active + Passive) of your own following the patterns given below.

Active Voice	Passive Voice
Is Hari helping them?	Are they being helped by Hari?
What do you want?	What is wanted by you?
Have you helped him?	Has he been helped by you?
Who has done this?	By whom has it been done?
Where have you kept the bags?	Where have the bags been kept by you?
What did Ravi buy?	What was bought by Ravi?
Who taught you Math?	By whom were you taught Math?
What were you writing?	What was being written by you?
Had Hari finished the story?	Had the story been finished by Hari?
When will you return my money?	When will my money be returned by you?